Praise for MENTAL FITNESS FOR LIFE

"Old age is not for sissies . . . mental fitness is a
physical fitness, say these experts. We are not
but rather liberated by it. It's a positive boo
best of the latest studies on aging plus some p.   to help
you maintain an active, flexible mind."

—*London Free Press*

If you ask anyone—whatever their age—what they are most
afraid of when they get older, they will probably say "losing it,"
and they assume memory will be the first to go. The "it" they
fear losing is mental fitness. Sandra Cusack and Wendy Thompson
disagree that aging and memory loss go hand in hand, and they
have evidence to prove it. They're out to change the world's
negative attitudes and beliefs about aging and memory loss, and
have created a program to keep people mentally fit.

—Liz Grogen, *Good Times Magazine*

"In their excellent book, Sandra Cusack and Wendy Thompson
have generously and intelligently provided us with exceedingly
useful information. Whatever your present age and current
beliefs, you can continue to improve and keep your mind fit and
enjoy life more than you ever dreamed."

—Dr. Marian Diamond, University of California at Berkeley

Mental Fitness for Life is a document of liberation for understanding
and enjoying the second half of life. The authors' thinking
represents a dramatic shift in the way we look at the process of
maturation and aging. This is an inspiring book."

—Dr. Arnold Scheibel, University of California, Los Angeles

MENTAL FITNESS FOR LIFE

7 STEPS TO HEALTHY AGING

REVISED EDITION

Sandra A. Cusack, Ph.D.

Wendy J.A. Thompson, M.A.

KEY PORTER 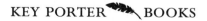 BOOKS

Library and Archives Canada Cataloguing in Publication

Cusack, Sandra, 1941–
    Mental fitness for life : 7 steps to healthy aging / Sandra A. Cusack and Wendy Thompson.—Rev. ed.

Includes bibliographical references and index.
ISBN 1-55263-682-8

    1. Cognition in old age.   2. Self-realization in old age.   I. Thompson, Wendy J. A.   II. Title.

BF724.85.C64C88 2004   158.1'084'6   C2004-907064-9

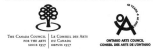

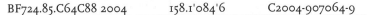

The Canada Council Le Conseil des Arts for the Arts du Canada since 1957 depuis 1957   ONTARIO ARTS COUNCIL CONSEIL DES ARTS DE L'ONTARIO

The publisher gratefully acknowledges the support of the Canada Council for the Arts and the Ontario Arts Council for its publishing program. We acknowledge the support of the Government of Ontario through the Ontario Media Development Corporation's Ontario Book Initiative.

We acknowledge the financial support of the Government of Canada through the Book Publishing Industry Development Program (BPIDP) for our publishing activities.

Key Porter Books Limited
Six Adelaide Street East, Tenth Floor
Toronto, Ontario
Canada M5C 1H6
www.keyporter.com

Text and Cover design: Ingrid Paulson
Electronic formatting: Heidy Lawrance Associates

Page 253 represents a continuation of this copyright page.

Printed and bound in Canada

05 06 07 08 09 6 5 4 3 2

This book is dedicated to the Mental Fitness Group at Century House, who demonstrated that age is more than a number and showed us that, at age 50 or 80 or 100,

Setting goals is worth it
Power thinking can be learned
Creativity is for everyone
Optimism creates health
Learning and memory can improve
Speaking your mind changes the world, inside and outside
Taking risks pays off
And living with purpose and passion keeps us fit—mentally, physically, emotionally, and spiritually.

To Joy Barkwill, manager of Century House, whose leadership, partnership, and friendship created the best possible environment for mental fitness research and programs. Thank you for being part of our dream.

CONTENTS

FOREWORD

What a privilege it is to write the foreword for this essential book on how to maintain an active brain for mental fitness throughout life, with emphasis on the quarter century after retirement. The authors believe that the data behind the new optimism on longevity is one of the most outstanding achievements of the 20th century, and I agree.

Life is a continuum from conception until death, with different stages of development and aging occurring simultaneously and continuously. To learn how to gain mental fitness at any age requires attention to and understanding of the brain's ability to respond to its ever-changing environment, but continued effort is essential as well.

The main question is "How do we get mentally fit and stay fit?" In their excellent book containing fact-filled examples, quotations, and humor, Sandra Cusack and Wendy Thompson, benefiting from years of experience studying and working in a 2,100-member seniors' center on the west coast of Canada, have generously and intelligently provided us with some exceedingly useful information. I thoroughly support, as do most people, their constant reminder of the importance of setting goals and maintaining a positive attitude at every stage of life; they give examples of how people achieve monumental tasks armed with such an attitude. In the long run, the only limitation in life is you yourself. Being positive certainly helps!

Maintaining an efficient memory to the end of life is a desire we all share. The authors offer a basic, clear discussion of different types of memory accompanied by several illustrated methods to achieve the desired objective of preserving a sound memory. Persistence and determination are essential. Stimulating activities and a good memory go hand in hand.

On a broader spectrum, the importance of having goals in life is stressed. How much more one can accomplish if physical, emotional, mental, and spiritual goals are developed and suitably modified when necessary. Directions are offered on how to achieve one's goals, such as making them measurable, identifying obstacles, identifying people to help reach one's goals, and planning a timeline.

Why not strive to become more vital, energetic, and beautiful both inside and out as we age? A list of successful people over 90 is provided to inspire us to continue to strive for excellence in our specific areas. The message of this book is "Whatever your present age and whatever your current beliefs, you can continue to improve, keep your mind fit and enjoy life more than you ever dreamed." What a concept to adopt from this time forward!

MARIAN C. DIAMOND, PH.D.
BERKELEY, CALIFORNIA

PREFACE

D o you exercise to stay in shape? Probably. Maybe you work out at a gym two or three times a week. You probably took Physical Education 101 in school, or was it Health and Personal Development 110? But we bet you didn't take "Mental Education 101" or "Mental Fitness 110" because there wasn't such a course. There is now, and you're on it. Few of us exercise to stay in shape mentally, but that is exactly what we are going to help you to do.

Our work in the research and development of mental fitness for older adults has been inspired by American researchers such as Marian Diamond at UC Berkeley, Arnold Scheibel at UCLA Medical Center, Ellen Langer at Harvard, Paul Davis Nussbaum at the University of Pittsburgh, K. Warner Schaie at Duke University, and David Snowdon at the University of Kentucky, who concur that lifelong learning and education have positive benefits for older adults. We now know that lifelong learning means different things to different people and encompasses all learning, formal and informal. Mental fitness is just as important as physical fitness, though less visible and more difficult to measure. In fact, mental fitness is the key to healthy and productive aging. But what is it and how do we exercise it?

Most people in middle and late adulthood today have grown up and are growing old with a general view of old age as a period of inevitable decline, and of old people as useless and burdens on society. Such negative attitudes and assumptions continue to haunt us, even when we know better. If you ask anyone, no matter how old they are, what they fear most about aging, they will probably say "losing it"—and they assume that memory is the first thing to go. What is "it" that they fear losing? "It" is precisely what this book is all about.

What exactly is "mental fitness," and how do we develop it? Seven years ago, we explored these two questions in an innovative community research project at Century House, a 2,100-member seniors' center on the west coast of Canada. We worked with a research group of 37 people aged 55 to 85 years (average age 73), representing a diversity of educational and occupational histories, ranging from people with a grade-school education to those with post-graduate degrees. Some had been retired for many years, some were newly retired, some recently laid off. Following ten months of intensive study and focus group discussion, we concluded that mental fitness was vital to healthy aging and it encompassed a number of skills that can be developed. Like physical fitness, it is a condition of optimal functioning that is achieved through regular exercise and a healthy lifestyle. Mental fitness includes setting personal goals, power thinking, creative thinking, learning and memory, speaking your mind, and a positive mental attitude characterized by optimism, mental flexibility, self-esteem, confidence, and willingness to risk.

Based on that research study and a working definition of mental fitness, an eight-week Mental Fitness for Life course was developed, and the first graduates (aged 63 to 83 years) completed an eight-week pilot program in 1996. (For this work, Century House subsequently received the 1997 Research Award presented by the National Institute of Seniors Centers, Washington, D.C.) The goal of the program was *mens sana in corpore sano* ("a healthy mind in a healthy body"). Our objectives were to exercise mental fitness skills and change attitudes and behavior. The program consisted of a series of eight all-day intensive workshops where participants learned how old attitudes and beliefs about declining mental abilities restricted their options for a vital old age. They learned how to change negative to positive beliefs that reflected their potential for growth, and they learned to speak the language of possibility. They learned how to think critically and creatively, to appreciate diversity and differing perspectives, to take risks, and to listen to each other with renewed respect.

Everyone who completed the pilot program benefited and all reported dramatic increases in their level of mental fitness and improved memory. More important than new knowledge and skills, participants gained new perspectives and more positive attitudes. As one woman said:

> *I have a newfound energy that is enabling me to think more clearly. I am doing things I never thought I could because of this excitement I have. I am striving for things I never thought I could achieve. Perhaps it was the limiting beliefs that held me back.*

And another said:

> *I used to believe that as we got older, our importance in the world diminished, our opinions were no longer sought, and our thoughts not respected. Now I know that it just isn't true.*

For this group of people, mental fitness has become a way of life. They continue to participate in a monthly seminar to exercise their minds. Their experience has been personally transformative: these people are more vital and active today than they were six years ago, and some are now in their 80s—one is 95. Each one is unique, but they have one thing in common: they are mentally fit for life.

Professionals in the field of aging are increasingly aware of the beneficial effects that education and learning have on general health as people age. As our research suggests, learning promotes health and is potentially transformative. While people involved in teaching and learning throughout life seem to have a higher level of mental fitness, research suggests that those who undertake something entirely different in their "third age" (that is, over 50), such as a new language or a musical instrument, have the edge. For example, you might expect university professors to be among the most mentally fit in Western societies. However, a professor who continues as professor emeritus after he or she retires may not get the kind of stimulation that is most beneficial. It may be time, as Monty Python used to say, for something completely different.

In this book you will discover how mentally fit you really are and what you can do to improve and maintain optimal mental and emotional health to the end of life. We have used seven years of experience in the research and development of an eight-week mental fitness program model as a basis for an individual program that will keep you mentally fit for life.

The chapters introduce the seven key mental fitness steps in the same order as the workshop sessions in the eight-week Mental Fitness for Life course. Each step begins with a warm-up consisting of quizzes and puzzles to get your brain limbered up. Puzzles stretch the brain and are extremely good for a mental workout. You can do them by yourself, but it is even better exercise to do them with a friend or a small group. It's a great idea for a party and there are plenty of puzzle books to choose from. We've included some favorite starter puzzles and quizzes, and we suggest you try these and then purchase your own puzzle book. As you work on solving them, your brain will begin to think in different ways, becoming more open and flexible. You'll be amazed at the different ways your brain will work for you—and how clever you really are. In solving the puzzles in this book, try to think out of the box, laterally, not linearly: try to get beyond old conventional ways of thinking, stretch your mind, and let your imagination run wild. Edward de Bono first coined the term "lateral thinking," which is a process of thinking that is different from the straightforward, logical way we normally think. When your brain starts to think "sideways" (laterally), you begin to solve problems in different ways—and not just the problems you encounter in a book. The results will translate into other areas of your life.

The seven key components of mental fitness are introduced with references to both research and practical experience. Wherever possible, our message is reinforced by the words of mental fitness program participants and sprinkled with words of wisdom from other noted authorities. Each chapter concludes with assignments—practical activities that we urge you to incorporate into your daily routine. No one ever told us that life would get easier as we got older. But it can get a whole lot more interesting and more fun if we are willing to work at things that are really important to us. And is there anything more important than you? Now, if anyone should ask if you are on a mental fitness program, you can tell them you are.

ACKNOWLEDGMENTS

We wish to thank our students, who confirmed our beliefs and taught us everything we know about mental fitness.

We are also very grateful to the distinguished American scholars whose seminal research provided the scientific foundation for our work: Paul Nussbaum, David Snowdon, Ellen Langer, K. Warner Schaie, Martin Seligman, and Gene Cohen.

For their encouragement and support, we thank our colleagues at Simon Fraser University: Gloria Gutman, Janice Baerg, Susan Jamieson-McLarnon, Yosef Wosk, and Bruce Whittlesea.

Thanks also to our agents at Seventh Avenue Literary Agency, Sally Harding and Robert Mackwood, and our editors at Key Porter, Clare McKeon and Meg Taylor.

Special thanks to Marian Diamond and Arne Scheibel, who are an inspiration to our work and serve as role models of healthy aging.

INTRODUCTION *to* MENTAL FITNESS

Mental Fitness is a state of mind in which we are open to enjoying our environment and the people in it, believing we have the capacity to be creative and imaginative. It is using our mental abilities to the fullest extent, taking risks, inquiring, questioning, and accepting other points of view, with a readiness to learn and grow and change.

—MENTAL FITNESS RESEARCH TEAM, NEW WESTMINSTER, B.C.

Around the globe, most spectacularly in the industrialized world, populations are aging. The mental fitness movement recognizes the growing potential in the older segment of society as a rich new source of energy just waiting to be harnessed.

In the early 21st century, we can expect to live 30 years beyond the traditional age of retirement. What will we do with this time? Learn how to grow old? That's a pretty dismal prospect, isn't it? The opposite extreme—being obsessed with looking and feeling young—is equally dangerous. That seems to be the preoccupation of many people who try to stop time at 40 or 50, or whatever they believe to be the height of their mental, emotional, and spiritual powers.

The good news is that we are, as a society, in the process of creating a new vision of the life course and the meaning of old age—one that celebrates longevity and focuses on realizing the untapped potential in older people for purposeful and vital living. The key life stages have been redefined: age 20 to 40 is now "young adulthood," 40 to 60 is considered middle age, and 60 to 80 is commonly referred to as "late adulthood." To be "old" or an "elder," one must be at least 80. There is more good news. Whereas decades of traditional research in aging supported a view of inevitable mental and physical decline, more recent research suggests that the mind can continue to grow and develop if it is stimulated and challenged.

You are about to embark on one of the most important and fascinating projects of your life—you are going to become happier and healthier than you have ever been before, the kind of person you would like to spend the rest of your life with. You probably never thought that you could be a great thinker at 70, 80, or 100, with the mental capacity to enjoy life to the fullest. In the language of mental fitness, this means

1. One who has confidence in his or her mental abilities
2. One who sets and achieves goals
3. One who is willing to take risks
4. One who is generally optimistic and has a positive outlook on life
5. One who expresses his or her uniqueness in creative and imaginative ways
6. One who is mentally flexible and listens to other points of view
7. One who is curious and interested in many topics, and finds joy in learning
8. One whose memory remains strong
9. One who speaks with clarity and conviction
10. One who is generally confident of his or her mental abilities

Isn't this precisely the kind of person you would choose to spend time with? Let's get to work. We have a lot of ground to cover.

Imagine a computer designed to satisfy your every desire and carry out your every command, a complex machine more powerful than anything a science fiction writer could imagine. You use it to store and retrieve every single piece of information collected over your entire lifetime. It remembers what you've read and your conversations with family, friends, and colleagues. It contains everything you ever wrote or even thought about. It weighs only about three pounds, but you must carry it around with you wherever you go. How careful would you be with this device? How gently would you treat it, maintain it, and protect it?

You have been entrusted with the care of one of the most extraordinary creations in the universe—the human brain. It is the home of your mind and your personality. It houses your memories, hopes, and dreams. Like a symphony orchestra, which depends upon each player to create a superb musical performance, your brain draws on all aspects of the mind: as each becomes tuned, performance improves, flows, and gives you a greater sense of purpose and passion than you could ever possibly imagine.

CHARTING YOUR COURSE *and* MEASURING YOUR PROGRESS

Mental fitness is about keeping the brain in top condition. First, you'll need information that you can use to chart your progress on the road to mental fitness. The trick is to be totally honest with yourself—in fact, a realistic awareness of your strengths and weaknesses is essential. Fill out the "How's Your Mental Fitness" quiz before you go any further. Then, when you've read through the book and engaged in various activities, you can take it again to rate your own progress and see what you have achieved.

⸘ HOW'S YOUR MENTAL FITNESS?

Rate yourself on a scale of 1 to 10 (10 being the highest rating).

_____   1. Confidence in your mental abilities

_____   2. Setting and achieving goals

_____   3. Willingness to take risks

_____   4. Optimism

_____   5. Creativity

_____   6. Mental flexibility

_____   7. Ability to learn new things

_____   8. Memory

_____   9. Ability to speak your mind clearly

_____ 10. Level of mental fitness

SELF-ASSESSMENT

Add up your score and rate yourself according to the following:

40–54   fair

55–69   good

70–84   very good

85–100 excellent

If your score is between 40 and 54, you will be delighted at the end of the program to find what progress you have made. If your score is between 55 and 69, be prepared to do some work and watch yourself improve. If it is 70 to 84, you are well on your way to enjoying a rich and fulfilling life—but don't be satisfied with the status quo. More than 85, and you are already an inspiration to others. We suggest shooting for 100. Like money in the bank, it's always good to have a reserve for yourself and some to give away to others.

Everybody believes that as we grow older we become slower, stiffer, more frail, and more disabled both physically and mentally. It's just the way life is. Right? It's common sense. It's the natural order. Everybody believes it's true. No one can go back in time to an age when they climbed trees, jumped fences, and ran the hundred-yard dash. Maybe if we never stopped doing those things, we'd still be able to. Who knows? Certainly, there are 90-year-olds who climb mountains. Maybe they never stopped, or maybe they just started. Chiang Hai Ding, a retired professor from Singapore, recently climbed Everest; now he is arranging to take his blind son on the next expedition.

No matter how stiff you have become or how many aches and pains you may have (and much of it may not be due simply to aging), it is never too late to get moving. We all need to keep climbing to the top of mountains—physically and mentally. When we rise to the challenge, somehow the energy that we need becomes available. And we gain a new view, a view that gives us a fresh perspective on our lives and what we can achieve through personal commitment and hard work. You will feel as though you are literally on top of the world. And consider this: if you're not climbing, you're slipping.

Here's the magic—we probably don't really want to jump fences anymore, but we all want to have plenty of energy for all the physical things we'd like to do. And we don't really want to memorize facts; we want to engage the world around us. The wonderful thing about aging in the 21st century is that we can learn and grow forever. New studies about the aging brain tell us to stop using aging as an excuse and get on with the rest of our lives.

No one would go to an exercise class once and say, "There, now I'm fit." In the same way, you need a well-designed fitness program for your mind, a program that has been tested and proven to work, that is guaranteed to wake up the energy inside you so that you can be the person you have always wanted to be.

No matter what age you are, 33 or 103, we all need to keep the mind healthy by challenging and stimulating it in a variety of ways. In the pages that follow, you'll read about the latest information and strategies to use daily or weekly for optimum performance of a healthy, fit mind. Like any effective training program, it takes effort to get and stay fit, but the rewards are incalculable. We used to believe that mental abilities automatically declined with age; now we know that's not true. We can actually improve our mental function and our memory to the end of life. We have seen it happen. We have experienced it ourselves. And you will, too.

> We are **not limited** by our old age; we are **liberated** by it.
>
> —STU MITTLEMAN

What is mental fitness? How do we get mentally fit? What effect does age have on mental function? How do we maintain our fitness? And how do we know when we are mentally fit? In other words, how do we measure it? What makes an extraordinary life? What's positive about aging? What do people fear most about getting older? And what steps can we take to ensure optimal mental functioning in our later years? These are the questions that everyone asks. The answers to these questions will help lay the foundation for healthy, happy aging.

New expectations, hopes, and dreams breathe purpose into life and fuel the passion that is so often missing. You will have an opportunity to set goals and achieve them. You have already achieved many goals in your life. What is important now is that as you age, you become all you can be—fulfilling your potential, using your talents, living each day to the fullest.

When you think about it, the way we think is the only thing we have control over, and the only thing we *need* to have control over. That's why working on your mental fitness is so important to healthy aging. Furthermore, you can control how much effort you put into your fitness program—no one is going to do it for you, and there is no instant, pill-popping way to fitness—mental or physical.

> The mind is a bit like a garden. **If it isn't fed** and cultivated, **weeds** will take it over.
> —ERVING G. HALL

This book focuses on adults over the age of 40. If you are 33, chances are pretty good that you will make it to 90 or 100. And you will get there (we guarantee it or your money back) healthier and happier when you are mentally fit, which you will be by the time you've finished this book and done your homework.

We'll introduce you to new studies on aging and the mind that paint an optimistic and empowering picture of aging. You'll meet the experts we've met across North America, through the literature and in person, all of whom shatter the myths of aging that most of us learned long ago. The mind knows no boundaries. You can become stronger and healthier by building on your strengths and the positive aspects of your life.

David Snowdon, professor of preventive medicine at the Sanders-Brown Center on Aging at the University of Kentucky, has been studying the nuns of Mankato in Minnesota for more than a decade. They have much to teach us about aging with grace, and how engagement in learning and teaching throughout life can keep the

> Aging is about **fire** and **rebirth**. It's about keeping passionate about someone and something and constantly **being reborn**.
> —PAUL TAGANYAKI

Most people say when you get old, you **have** **to** give things up. I say you get old **because** you give things up.

—SENATOR THEODORE GREEN OF RHODE ISLAND, WHO SERVED IN THE U.S. SENATE UNTIL HE WAS 94

brain active well into old age. The sisters of Mankato lead intellectually challenging lives; we are beginning to learn how stimulating the mind with mental exercise causes brain cells, or neurons, to branch wildly. These women also do not seem to suffer from dementia, Alzheimer's, and other debilitating brain diseases as early or as severely as the general population. As David Snowdon writes,

The School Sisters of Notre Dame have shown me that old age is not something to fear and revile. It can be a time of promise and renewal, of watching with a knowing eye, of accepting the lessons that life has taught and, if possible, passing them on to the generations that follow. What I have learned from the sisters—many of whom remain mentally robust after a century of life—is . . . hope for the future.

You will unleash great inner power when you begin to think seriously about mental fitness and put it into action. Many people live far below their potential and many are unaware of the power of a healthy, fit mind. We hold beliefs that prevent us from living lives we only dream about. In this book you will learn to recognize those limiting beliefs and learn how to eliminate them. We can keep the brain healthy as we age by feeding it regularly. The mind is like a garden that can be cultivated to bear fruit, and that's what mental fitness is—getting rid of the weeds and cultivating the fruit.

But before we launch you on your program, let's do a quick review of the outdated research and demonstrate why it's no longer either helpful or correct.

AGING *and* MENTAL ABILITIES:
A BRIEF REVIEW *of* RESEARCH

During the 1960s and 70s, the question most often addressed in the studies was whether older adults were capable of functioning at the same level as younger people. The traditional approach to memory research assumed that mental functioning declined with age, and researchers generally focused on tasks that involved learning and memory. These studies showed that older people functioned at a lower level on a variety of tasks in many different situations.

We know now that much of that research was flawed. Findings suggest two important features discriminated against "the elderly" and they are (1) the speed of the response and (2) meaningfulness of the task. In other words, if you give older people more time and give them a task that interests them, they do just as well as anyone else. It is what you do with that information that is important. For example, if you are mentally fit and optimistic, you may interpret that information as follows: younger people are able to absorb meaningless information quickly, whereas older people are more discriminating and selective and conserve their energy for more important things. Remember, everything depends on the spin you give it. Furthermore, wouldn't we all, young and old, like to slow things down a bit? Let's take our cue from older people, so that everyone can contribute. Those early studies regarding mental abilities and aging reinforced the notion that memory will get worse and it's all downhill once you hit 50. Not anymore.

> The brain has muscles for thinking as the legs have muscles for walking.
>
> —J.O. DE LA METTRIE, AUTHOR OF *L'HOMME MACHINE*, 1748

During the past decade, a more optimistic view has emerged: aging does not mean inevitable decline. Evidence is accumulating that the brain works a lot like a muscle—the harder you use it, the more it grows. For decades scientists have believed that the brain was more or less fixed by adolescence and did not have much flexibility to develop in adulthood. We have now discovered that the human brain has the capacity to change and adapt well into old age.

During the 1960s, Dr. Marian Diamond, professor of anatomy in the Department of Integrative Biology at the University of California at Berkeley, began her groundbreaking rat studies, which concluded that mental stimulation prolongs life. While physical abilities may diminish, the mind will not—provided it is stimulated and challenged (witness David Snowdon's research with the nuns of Mankato). Research on the aging brain supports the possibilities for mental and psychological growth and development to the end of life.

The great American feminist Betty Friedan cited two factors that predicted a longer life: not smoking, and engaging in complex social and mental activities. Friedan found that those who engage in purposeful activity (and have social connections other than family) live longer, and they also enjoy a better quality of life. Developing the mind can slow down or even reverse physical changes typically associated with aging. Developing the mind is, indeed, the key to vital aging.

MENTAL FITNESS and HEALTHY AGING

What is the relationship between an active mind and healthy aging? In the literature today, people use terms like "mental fitness" (Allen D. Bragdon) and "mental aerobics" (Marge Engelman). The American Society on Aging has developed a "Mindalert Program," with an annual awards competition. When we first began to explore the research ten years ago, looking for hints regarding how to define mental fitness, we found a number of researchers with important things to say about the relationship between an active mind and healthy aging, and the basic components of a mental fitness program. We were guided by their research, and our work in turn helped to confirm these findings throughout the 1990s.

An American researcher by the name of Irene Burnside explored the meaning of health and fitness and well-being for older women, and she developed a framework for "fitness" with four separate categories: physical fitness, intellectual fitness, social fitness, and "purpose" fitness. Purpose fitness she describes as having a healthy self-esteem and control over one's life. Furthermore, physical health is not as important to women in later life as their attitude toward their own health problems and their ability to survive. Developing one's ability to cope with change and loss may lead to a positive attitude—and it is this positive attitude and the sense of self-esteem that comes from having a sense of personal control over one's life that are most critical to healthy aging.

David Featherman and his colleagues at the Institute for Social Research, University of Michigan, define successful aging as effectively meeting the many challenges life presents, which can be enhanced by learning to plan. Developing the mind leads to better health if it includes developing coping skills, a positive attitude, and making plans for the future (setting personal goals). Featherman's research provides more evidence for including goal setting, a sense of purpose, and a positive attitude as part of overall mental fitness.

Both Burnside and Featherman support the notion that being mentally fit is associated with better health. However, we could find no strong evidence in the research literature of a positive relationship between mental attitude or a sense of purpose in life and general health. An American group, Morris A. Okun and colleagues at Arizona State, reviewed all the research literature on learning and health prior to the mid-1980s and reported that, while the number of educational programs for older adults was increasing dramatically, there was still no experimental evidence of the impact of education on

standard measures of health. We do know that older adults experience increased well-being by participating in such programs. Indeed,
many educational programs for older adults are created to enhance
well-being. Yet we could find no solid evidence that this is true, so we
set about gathering our own evidence, inspired by Deepak Chopra
and Harvard researcher Ellen Langer.

There is now a widely accepted belief that the mind, body, and
spirit are intimately connected. Deepak Chopra, M.D., has written
extensively about the body–mind connection, integrating Western
medicine and Eastern mysticism, and providing new insights about
the power of the mind over the body. He claims that just as we in
Western societies learn to grow old, we can *reverse* the effects of age
by the power of the mind.

> *No one gave us any limitations on the patterns of intelligence we*
> *can make, change, blend, expand, and inhabit. Life is a field of*
> *unlimited possibilities. Such is the glory of total flexibility in the*
> *human nervous system. . . . The current scientific wisdom holds*
> *that aging is a complicated, poorly understood area. The study of*
> *old age has become a specialization only since the 1950s. The*
> *major advance in the field has been to document that healthy*
> *people do not have to deteriorate automatically as they grow*
> *older, a point that has been made for centuries without data*
> *banks. Officially, gerontology recognizes no means to reverse or*
> *retard the aging process—a rather stringent position, when you*
> *consider that aging has not even been adequately defined. The*
> *rishis (Eastern mystics) would counter by saying that science has*
> *failed to reach the level of awareness where aging can be defeated.*

Chopra reports dramatic evidence, supported by research, that
the physical aspects of age can be altered by the power of the mind.

The great sage Shankara who towers over the whole tradition of Indian philosophy once wrote, "People grow old and die because they see other people growing old and dying." Shankara's seemingly strange idea that we grow old because we watch others grow old may well be true.

We discovered an ingenious study by Dr. Ellen Langer and her associates at Harvard University that was conducted in the late 1970s, long before anyone began to use the term "mental fitness." Langer and her team were testing whether aging was as irreversible as everyone believed it to be. Langer's team had its doubts; they suspected that aging itself might be a creation of the mind, which the mind can, in fact, reverse.

To test this possibility, they first placed a newspaper ad in a Boston daily asking for men seventy-five and older who would be willing to go on a week's vacation, all expenses paid. A group of suitable volunteers was chosen, placed in a van, and whisked off to a luxurious retreat on ten acres of secluded woodland in the New England countryside.

When they arrived at this isolated setting, the men were met with a duplicate of daily life as it existed twenty years earlier. Instead of magazines from 1979, the reading tables held issues of Life *and the* Saturday Evening Post *from 1959. The radio played music from that year, and group discussions centered on the politics and celebrities of the era. A taped address from President Eisenhower was played, followed by the film* Anatomy of a Murder, *which won the Academy Award in 1959. Besides these props, every effort was made to center each person on how he felt, looked, talked, and acted when he was twenty years younger.*

The group had to speak exclusively in the present tense as if 1959 were today, and their references to family, friends, and jobs could not go beyond that year. Their middle-aged children were still at home or just going to college; their careers were in full swing. Each person had submitted a picture of himself taken twenty years before; these were used to introduce each one to the group.

While this week of make-believe went on, a control group of men over seventy-five also talked about the events of 1959, but using the past tense instead of the present. Castro, Mickey Mantle, Eisenhower, and Marilyn Monroe were allowed to have their real futures. The radio played 1979 music, the magazines carried the latest news, and the films were current releases.

Before, during, and after the retreat, Langer measured each man for signs of aging. For the members of the 1959 group, to a remarkable extent these measurements actually went backward in time over the one-week period. The men began to improve in memory and manual dexterity. They were more active and self-sufficient (instead of waiting to be helped, for example, they took their food and cleared the tables by themselves).

Some such changes might be expected in any older person enjoying himself on vacation. However, traits that are definitely considered irreversible signs of aging also started to turn around. Independent judges looked at before-and-after pictures of the men and rated them three years younger in appearance. Hand measurements showed that their fingers had actually lengthened and gained back some of the flexibility in their joints. The group could sit taller in their chairs, had a stronger hand grip, and could even see and hear better. The control group also exhibited some of these changes but to a smaller degree, and in some measures, such as manual dexterity and finger length, they had even declined over the week.

In her intriguing book *Mindfulness*, Langer attributes some of these reversals to the fact that the men were given more control over their lives than they enjoyed at home. They were treated like anyone in his mid-50s, who would naturally carry his own suitcase or select his own food for dinner. Their opinions were valued in group discussions, and it was assumed that they

You can't climb uphill if you are thinking downhill thoughts.

were mentally vigorous, an assumption probably not made about them in everyday life. In this way they moved from a mindless existence to one that is "mindful," Langer's term for living with alertness, openness to new ideas, and mental vigor. Langer's term "mindfulness" is similar to the attitude of mind of one who is mentally fit. Mental fitness goes beyond vigor, flexibility, and alertness to encompass a range of skills and abilities and, most importantly, an attitude of optimism.

BUILDING BRAIN POWER

We can train the brain not just to maintain its present level of function but to improve mental function as we age. New research tells us that if we don't ever want to feel like we're not as sharp or as mentally fit as we used to be, we just need to exercise those skills and adopt a more positive and flexible attitude toward life.

Dr. K. Warner Schaie at Duke University is in the forefront of intervention research. Two hundred and twenty-nine men and women (aged 65 and over) were tutored for five hours in skills they seemed to be losing—the two skills chosen were "spatial orientation" (which is related to reading maps and finding your way in the external world) and "inductive reasoning" (which refers to logical analysis). "When given a booster course and tested seven

The **memory** capacity of an ordinary human mind is **fabulous**. We may not consider ourselves particularly adept at remembering **technical data** . . . but consider how many faces we can recognize, how many names call up some past incident, how many words we can spell and define. . . . It is estimated that in a **lifetime**, a brain can store 1,000,000,000,000,000 (a million billion) **"bits"** of information.

—ISAAC ASIMOV

years later, their skills were still sharp . . . getting tutored isn't necessary . . . any mental exercise that you do on your own should benefit your brainpower, and the more the better."

Arnold Scheibel of the UCLA Medical School concurs: "Research in the brain sciences has shown with increasing clarity that our brain maintains some degree of plasticity till the very end of life and even more important, that each of us has the ability to 'take our brains in hand.'" While few people see old age as a time to continue learning, science is beginning to demonstrate that the more we challenge the brain, the better we are able to face the very real mental and emotional challenges of the later years.

The message is loud and clear. You can keep your brain in shape by feeding and working it. People commonly experience forgetfulness and lack of concentration and assume that is part of old age. New research suggests that we can keep the brain active. We are born with a certain number of brain cells. When cells are used, they spread like the branches of a tree. The more branches, or dendrites, you have, the more brain power you have. Just as trees need water and sun, dendrites need stimulation. People age more successfully, think better, and don't feel as old if they keep their minds active. People who benefit from mental stimulation, who think creatively, do better in old age. Those with mundane jobs have to seek out mental stimulation elsewhere. Think of it as a retirement investment. Along with financial planning, potential retirees would do well to focus on planning a personal mental fitness program that would exercise mental abilities, give them a jump-start, and set them on a course of discovering their personal "fountain of age."

Current research tells us that growth and development of the mind can continue to the end of life. Unfortunately, decline in mental abilities with age is considered normal. Lowered expectations serve as self-fulfilling prophecies. Why should we accept the status quo?

Here goes—this is your first exercise. It's fun, and you will be surprised at some of the answers. Go ahead, try your luck. The answers are in "Clues and Answers," page 239 (no peeking!).

♻ BRAIN TEASER

1. How long did the Hundred Years War last?
2. Which country makes Panama hats?
3. From which animal do we get catgut?
4. In which month do Russians celebrate the October Revolution?
5. What is a camel's hair brush made of?
6. The Canary Islands in the Pacific are named after what animal?
7. What was King George VI's first name?
8. What color is a purple finch?
9. Where are Chinese gooseberries from?
10. How long did the Thirty Years War last?

In the chapters that follow, you'll be launched on your own mental fitness program. Goal Setting will give your life a focused purpose. Power Thinking will teach you new and powerful ways of thinking. Creativity is limitless, depending only on how far you want to get out of the box. Positive Mental Attitude will change your life forever, giving you the emotional health you need to create optimal mental and physical health. Memory can improve as you age, through lifelong learning. Speaking Your Mind will give you the voice you've always wanted to express yourself and live your dreams.

BENEFITS *of* MENTAL FITNESS *for* LIFE

Here is how this program will work for you—if you do the work—in the words of participants:

- "I used to believe the golden years were fool's gold. After being in the program, I now believe the golden years are whatever you want to create for yourself."
- "The program is thought-provoking, stimulating, and fun. More than ever before, I actively explored my mind."
- "It challenged me in every area of my life, but more than that—it gave me a future to think about and believe in."
- "Finding out what your brain is capable of learning and retaining is amazing. Now I give my brain a daily workout and I can almost hear those dendrites growing."
- "I discovered that my brain had only been sleeping, not slipping."
- "Solving brain puzzles is not only fun, not only a new way to entertain yourself, but it has given me confidence in my mental powers—more confidence than I ever had before."

OVERVIEW *of the* 7 STEPS

STEP 1: GOAL SETTING

In Step 1, we will explore why it is important to set goals and we'll look at some of the reasons people don't set them. We will introduce you to activities that will develop your skill at setting goals and achieving them. Achieving goals depends in large part on your motivation and desire. Desire and commitment will be generated in the following ways:

- By identifying those things that have value in life
- By developing personal goals using a 10-step process
- By convincing yourself that you can set achievable goals
- By supporting and encouraging you in achieving goals

STEP 2: POWER THINKING

Step 2 explores power thinking as a process and a skill. Simply put, power thinking means out with the old beliefs and in with the new. This process involves the following steps:

1. Identifying limiting beliefs
2. Challenging them
3. Learning to think in new ways
4. Replacing limiting beliefs with beliefs that serve you well

We will raise your awareness and develop critical thinking skills by

- Identifying your personal fears about old age and underlying beliefs
- Convincing you of the power of your personal belief system

- Helping you to recognize statements based on a limiting belief (to erase the belief from your mind)
- Helping you to change the language of limiting beliefs to the language of limitless possibility

STEP 3: **CREATIVITY**

The focus in Step 3 is creative thinking. New research suggests that people can develop their creativity well into later life. Participants in our mental fitness classes say they became more creative than they used to be because they no longer thought of creativity as being restricted to artistic expression. It became easier for them to think "out of the box"—to think and act in radically different ways.

STEP 4: **POSITIVE MENTAL ATTITUDE**

In Step 4, we discuss the importance of a positive mental attitude and the new research that indicates positive attitudes can be learned. You will complete an optimism test and discover how to become more optimistic.

STEP 5: **MEMORY AND LEARNING**

While everyone is concerned about memory, few appreciate the intimate connection between learning and memory that the following phrase characterizes: "If you can't remember something, you probably never learned it." Learning new things causes the dendrites to grow and branch wildly, improving brain power. Research suggests that most benefits come from learning something that is quite different from what has been learned in the past. For example, learning a new language has been shown to have great benefit. You will gain tips and strategies for improving your ability to learn new information.

STEP 6: **SPEAKING YOUR MIND**

In Step 6, we will give you the encouragement you need to use your newfound mental fitness skills and to speak your mind more honestly and eloquently—to make a difference in the world.

STEP 7: **MENTALLY FIT FOR LIFE**

The final chapter focuses on achieving personal goals, strategies for maintaining mental fitness, and creating a vision of what you plan to do from now on and the rest of your life: "Thirty things to do before I die."

So, let's get on with it. What would you *really* like to do with the rest of your life?

STEP 1

GOAL SETTING:
FINDING *Your* PURPOSE *and* PASSION

Every person, when they get quiet,
when they become desperately honest with themselves, is capable
of uttering profound truths.
We all derive from the same source.
There is no mystery about the origin of creation.
We are all part of creation,
all kings, all queens, all poets, all musicians;
we have only to open up, only to
discover what is already there.

—HENRY MILLER

REFLECTIONS *on* GOAL SETTING

My first goal was at age 57 and it was to prepare for old age, and I'm still working on it. —Bob Wain, age 84

Most of us never thought about goals until we graduated from school. When the principal asked me what I was going to be, I told him I didn't want to be a secretary, and his response was "That's too bad." —Jean Martinuik, age 64

I grew up in a different era. Coming through the Depression, we were lucky to have a roof over our heads. I wanted to be a nurse, but that was a dream. All you really wanted to do was to survive, so I became a secretary. —Freda Hogg, age 83

GOAL SETTING *and* ACHIEVEMENT

This is where the program begins. It is also where a more successful, productive, meaningful, healthy, and happy life begins.

In this chapter we discuss why goal setting is so important. We explore why some people don't set goals, and we look at goal setting in later life. Our review of the research touches briefly on important studies from the 1950s to the 1970s that suggest that the common myths regarding aging and setting goals have no basis in fact. We examine the evidence showing that goal setting keeps the mind fit.

You will be introduced to the 10-step process for setting and achieving goals, and you'll be challenged to complete activities that will change your life. Before going further, here are some brain teasers that will give your mind a good workout.

⌕ MENTAL FITNESS WARM-UP

After reading each question—and they are meant to tease you—stop and think hard. Don't automatically say the answer. There is a twist, so let your mind search through its pathways to the right answer.

1. Why are 1990 American dollar bills worth more than 1989 American dollar bills?
2. Is there a fourth of July in England?
3. How many animals of each sex did Moses take on the ark?
4. A clerk in the butcher shop is 5 feet, 10 inches tall. What does he weigh?
5. How many 2-cent stamps are there in a dozen?
6. Overheard: "I eat what I can and I can what I can't." What does that mean?
7. Avoiding the Train: A man was walking along a railway track when he spotted an express train speeding toward him. To avoid it, he jumped off the track, but before he jumped he ran ten feet toward the train. Why?
8. A man left home one day and made three left turns and met a man with a mask on. What was the first man's profession?

(Answers in "Clues and Answers," page 239.)

Aging is about discovering new beginnings and is now defined as growing and developing. Perhaps the major goal of every life is to realize dreams and develop our full potential in every aspect of our lives. In order to grow and develop and reach our full potential, we need to set goals and achieve them. It's as simple as that, but not easy to do unless you know how.

> To achieve **happiness, we should make certain that we are never without** an **important goal.**
> —EARL NIGHTINGALE

People have written about setting and achieving goals for decades. Goals are the foundation of most of what we have accomplished, and setting them motivates us in a way that nothing else can. Personal and professional achievement at any level is served best by setting goals and planning how to achieve them. How on earth can you get where you are going if you don't have a road map?

The Value of Goals

In 1953, a historic study was conducted at Yale University with the senior graduating class. The students were surveyed with a variety of questions, one of which was "Do you have goals and have you made plans for achieving them?" Results showed that only 3 percent of the graduating class, one of the most favored groups graduating from a prestigious university in America, had goals.

These same students were surveyed 20 years later and one of the many questions was "How much money are you worth today compared to what you were worth in 1953?" Results showed that the 3 percent who set goals at the beginning of their careers were worth more in financial terms than the entire remaining 97 percent put together. Of course, the point is not how much money we have or how many material possessions we have accumulated. As a matter of fact, experts tell us that only 3 percent of the population have clear goals and the plans for their accomplishment.

It doesn't take any specific brain power to create dreams and action plans—anyone at any age can do that. However, goal setting is a critical skill that must be learned and then applied if we want to be truly successful in life and reach our full human potential. Goal setting has rarely been a focus for personal development work with people aged over 50. That's why we have included the goals workshop in this book.

> Something we were withholding made us weak. Until we found it was ourselves.
>
> —ROBERT FROST

If you want something different, one of the best ways to get it is to create your own research project. The topic—*you*. People take courses, go to night school, believe in life-long learning, and get degrees in every conceivable area of learning. The most important area to gain expertise in is yourself. For results that improve the quality of life and to feel a sense of worth and success, we need to study ourselves. What makes us tick? What makes us sick? What makes us feel satisfied at the end of the day? What do we really want? Who do we want to be?

> *To most [people] there should come a time for shifting harness, for lightening the load one way and adjusting it for greater effort in another. This is the time for the second career. The new career may bring in little or no money; it may be concerned only with good works. It may, on the other hand, bring in support that is much needed. It can be a delight to [everyone] who comes at last to a well-earned job instead of a well-earned rest. It can be, too, what society needs most from [them].*
>
> —WILDER PENFIELD

"If you really want to live a long and healthy life," said Hans Selye, the international expert on stress, "do things that excite you, that you are passionate about." Do not retire (at least not from life)—get involved in projects that contribute and bless other people's lives.

Goals—setting them and achieving them—serve us in myriad ways. They create a sense of purpose; they create a sense of self-worth and a willingness to explore opportunities to become excellent. Everyone has the potential to excel in some area. Goals help us find and then explore what we love to do, they enable us to be in control of the constant change in life. Setting goals is like keeping our hands on the steering wheel of life. We can control our goals and we can choose the direction we want to focus our efforts on.

You cannot discover new oceans unless you have the courage to lose sight of the shore.

You are where you are as a result of what you have been thinking and doing for the past 10, 20, 30, 40, 50, 60, 70 years . . .

If you want more than you now have, you need to start thinking and doing something different or you will continue to have more of the same!

Failure is not necessarily missing the target, but aiming too low.

What would you dare to attempt if you believed it was impossible to fail? What would you dare to attempt if you believed you would succeed?

The Reasons People Do Not Set Goals

Why don't people set goals? The only time that most people are really happy is when they have a goal. The only time we are fully alive is

It is a **funny thing** about life; if you refuse to **accept anything** but the best, you very **often get it.**

—SOMERSET MAUGHAM

when we are involved in something that is important to us. Better still, something we are passionate about. As Betty Friedan, author of *The Fountain of Age*, says, we all need projects and a sense of purpose in our lives. This is what gives us a sense of direction, recognition, and significance.

Despite this, there are many reasons people don't set goals. As you read them, see if any apply to you. The first reason people don't set goals is that they don't realize the importance of having a purpose. Maybe you haven't thought about goals, or they were never discussed in your family. No one ever suggested that you write them down. Perhaps you felt it was selfish to think or dream of things for yourself; you may have helped your spouse or friends fulfill their goals. But these reasons don't need to apply anymore. Remember, this research project is about *you*.

The second reason people don't set goals is because they don't know how. If this applies to you, no one's blaming you. There wasn't Goal Setting 101 for any of us. Now there is.

Big goals can create a fear of **failure.** Lack of goals **guarantees** it.

The third reason people don't set goals is the fear of rejection. Experts give us various ways of dealing with this one, but in a nutshell, here's what we found works best. Keep your goals confidential—that is, away from anyone who will criticize them or laugh at them. Remember when you were a kid and you said you wanted to be a fireman or an astronaut, and someone said to you, "You must be kidding. Quit daydreaming! How about a nurse or a secretary?" On the other hand, by all means share your goals with people who will encourage and support whatever it is you want to do or become. If you want to climb Mount Everest or conduct an orchestra or learn a new language or write a book or learn to draw—you can do it. Go for it. Tell the people who will support you. Give them regular progress reports. Ask them to give you the help you need.

> Failure will **never overtake me** if my **desire** to succeed is **strong** enough.
>
> —OG MANDINO

The fourth reason people don't set goals is fear of failure. In fact, this is the number one reason people fail in life. They have messages in their head that say, "I can't. I'm not good enough. I might be embarrassed if I try. There's a good chance that I'll fail, and I already feel like a failure." The major issue here is understanding failure. The classic antidote to the fear of failure is the story of Thomas Edison, who was one of the greatest failures of all time. He failed thousands of times in trying to find a filament for the electric light bulb; this became known as "Edison's folly." When a reporter asked Edison why he persisted in spending his time and money after he kept failing, Edison replied, "I haven't failed at all. I have successfully discovered five thousand ways that will not work. And now I'm five thousand ways closer to what *will* work." And he did finally succeed and lit the world.

The fifth reason people don't set goals is they think they are too old. They spend too much time thinking and talking of the past. They don't spend enough time living in the present, enjoying what they have, and planning for their future. The vast majority of older people have very long futures—or at the very least, much longer than they think they have.

Goal setting is fundamental to a feeling of well-being. We can create the future when we achieve goals. It is the goals in our lives—personal and career goals—that drive success. We are going to help you achieve goals in the 10-step process that really works.

Everyone dreams;
but not equally.
Those who dream by night
in the dusty recesses
of their minds
wake in the day
to find that it was vanity:
but the dreamers of the day
are dangerous,
for they may act their dream
with open eyes;
to make it possible.

—T.E. LAWRENCE

Goal Setting in Later Life

As people age, goals and dreams are talked about less and less; they seldom are referred to in books for older people, because many believe it's too late to set goals. Older people often believe that their future is not sufficiently long to set goals, and they have more or less done it all. Furthermore, many have accomplished and accumulated a lot without consciously setting goals.

With few exceptions, the prevailing attitude among older people and at every level of society is still that the third age or retirement phase (which can begin as young as 50) is the time to relax, play golf, and travel. In fact, tourism is now the biggest industry in the world. And tour companies take care of *everything* right down to the last detail—when to get up, when to pack your bag, when to eat, when to get on the bus, how much to tip the driver. But we know that's not all older people want,

The first two letters of goal are "go."

nor is it the only thing they do in retirement—nor is it what makes for a healthy old age.

Relaxing and spending time with family are worthy activities, but they are not necessarily what make us feel fulfilled, and they don't always bring the sense of deep meaning that leads to greater happiness and quality of life. We are simply saying that there is so much more.

> When one door closes, another opens; but we often look so long and so regretfully upon the closed door that we do not see the one which has opened for us.
>
> —ALEXANDER GRAHAM BELL

Some people actually spend time looking backward, thinking and dwelling on the past because it's easier to do that than try to figure out where they want to go. By the end of this chapter, we want to convince you of the importance of setting goals and to provide strategies and steps that you can take to enable you, no matter how old you are, to create the health and happiness we all want and desire.

Setting goals is different for older people. They have years and years of experience, which informs their judgments and opinions—positive and negative beliefs and assumptions about various aspects of their lives and the world. Unfortunately, many have developed negative beliefs about themselves and their abilities as they age and move into the retirement phase of life. Many have developed negative beliefs about aging in general and have negative expectations about their own aging. Negative beliefs keep people stuck, keep them from developing and achieving results. (Step 2 is devoted to examining our beliefs and teaches how

> Dare mighty things, even though checkered with failure, rather than to rank with those gray souls that know neither victory nor defeat.
>
> —THEODORE ROOSEVELT

to eradicate any negative ones, turning them into empowering beliefs that unlock our potential.)

The vast majority of people over 50 today have never formally worked on goal setting. Until the 1990s, goal-setting workshops weren't widely available. Now almost every book on personal and professional development has chapters on setting goals and getting results, and courses are available and accessible to everyone through professional development and continuing education programs.

Goal setting is a process for getting where you want to go. Some people have had goals throughout their lives; others never set goals—they survived by living from challenge to challenge, from day to day, responding to what was expected of them. Goal setting is not something they may have practiced throughout their earlier years, and they may need to experience what a dynamic tool it is for getting things done.

> What lies **behind** us and what lies **before** us are tiny matters, compared to what **lies** within us.
>
> —OLIVER WENDELL HOLMES

We will introduce you to goal setting as a 10-step process for getting where you want to go. Goals are like maps—they keep you on course and help you to clarify what is important in your life. Goals are also like magnets—they attract things and people that help to get them accomplished. Accomplishing a goal that you have set for yourself feels good and gives you the confidence to achieve more than you ever thought you could.

When they were younger, most older people today were too busy earning a living to ever think about goals—some barely survived during the Depression. Many never had the time or the will to "shape their own future." But now they do. Whenever the opportunity comes, seize it and get busy.

Shape Your Own Vision

To be truly successful you must examine your talents
And form an exact picture of what you want to be.
It's like a hook in your brain that draws you forward
Because you're reeled in by your own vision.

Few people are capable of making a difference in the world,
But nearly everyone can perform at an exceptional level
If he or she chooses a field that best expresses
Their knowledge, talent, drive, and interest.

Start to think very clearly about what it is
At the center of your life
You want to be or do
And then let nothing stand in your way.

Once you have shaped that vision
You are no longer at the mercy of random events.

Those who pursue a vision
Must assume responsibility and take risks.
The risks are facing an inner dialogue,
Being alone, and making decisions.
The responsibility is to maintain courage,
Intensity, skill, and dedication.

The safest thing in the world is to do nothing.
There's no way that making things happen is easy.
Final success comes not from status and wealth
But from making a contribution to society.

These words were spoken to a high school graduating class by Maurice Gibbons, former professor of education at Simon Fraser University, but the words speak to anyone at any age who is embarking on a new phase of life—a phase of life that can be characterized by energy and vitality, purpose and passion, and a desire to be the best you can be. That is what living and aging is all about.

Let's take a look at what the research literature has to say about goal setting and achieving and aging. It is always useful to have a historical perspective, because it often provides new insights and a deeper understanding of the topic. We asked participants in the mental fitness program, "What is different about setting goals when you are older?" This is what they had to say:

- We don't have any limitations—so we can go for it.
- We have more time to do what we want to.
- When you have a goal, it helps you focus on the future.
- It's easy to fritter away your time—and so it's very important that older people set goals.
- The happiest people are focused in the moment and working toward the future.
- With unstructured time, you need to structure your day. I start at 5:30 a.m. with a very tight schedule—I never got up that early when I was working.
- If you don't have a purpose, you do nothing.
- It is more important to set goals, because we have less time left.
- When you are retired from work, you lose self-worth—so you have to have a goal for self-esteem.
- I enjoyed the first year after retirement. Now that has passed and this course is just what I need. I am aware of the loss of richness of roles. At this time, I have a choice—multiple roles are gone.

Goal setting is arguably the most important component of getting mentally fit, because it is where we identify what is really important to us—where we find a sense of meaning and purpose in life—and then develop the skills and resources for achieving them. We use power thinking to get rid of negative beliefs that may be preventing us from achieving our goals. We use creativity to express our unique talents and skills, and to create our own future as older people in an aging world—thus unleashing energy and vitality. We work on a positive mental attitude to give us hope for the future. We use strategies to improve learning and memory so that we remain confident in our ability to learn and grow. We speak out with clarity about what really matters. Finally, we establish a program to ensure that we are mentally fit for life. All this in the interest of achieving our goals.

> No matter how difficult the past, you can always begin again today.

Goal setting is a thread that runs through every workshop in the Mental Fitness for Life program. The goals can be big; they can be small; they can be personal; they can be professional. They include short-term goals such as quitting smoking, losing weight, keeping a journal, exploring creativity through the arts, developing a more positive attitude, memorizing poetry, researching the family tree.

> When you cease to make a contribution, you begin to die.
>
> —ELEANOR ROOSEVELT

Goals can also be related to one's mission in life, like the School Sisters of Notre Dame whose mission is helping others to live life fully through teaching and learning.

Wilder Penfield, the Canadian surgeon who is known for his pioneering brain research in the 1950s, was ahead of his time—he rejected the notion of retirement altogether. Following a career as a brain researcher, Penfield became a public speaker. The speech that catapulted him into public consciousness was "Pseudo-Senility: Osler's Dictum Reconsidered." It was a challenge to the whole notion of old age and retirement. In his address, he quoted William Osler's final address as retiring director of Johns Hopkins Medical School at the turn of the 20th century. Osler is quoted as saying:

> I have two fixed ideas. The first is the comparative uselessness of men above forty years of age. . . . My second fixed idea is the uselessness of men above sixty years of age, and the incalculable benefit it would be in commercial, political and in professional life if, as a matter of course, men stopped work at this age.

Fifty-five years after Osler's address, Penfield went on to describe how the newspapers had picked it up and run headlines saying "MEN USELESS AFTER FORTY" and "SHOULD BE CHLORO-FORMED AT SIXTY." "Oslerizing the aged" entered common speech, and in St. Louis a man of 60 killed himself, leaving an empty chloroform bottle and newspaper clippings referring to Osler's speech on the bed beside him.

This became a platform for Wilder Penfield's strong contrary views and his second career as a public speaker. He is quoted:

> Let me describe to you the evolution of a little-recognized disease. It is a psychological malady, which we might name pseudo-senility. A worthy citizen employed in business, for example, . . . reaches his time of statutory retirement. Some colleague, who happens to have a larger bank account of unspent

years, comes to him and gives him a gold watch and tells him
to take a well-earned rest. That man, who yesterday was busy
and capable of contributing something of value, now stays
home. He mows the lawn and carries out the garbage for his
wife while he thinks about his future. When he is well-behaved
she lets him wash the dishes. He notices that his recent memory
is not as good as it was when he was younger, although distant
memory is good enough. In a little while, people begin to say,
behind his back of course: "He's going to pieces, poor fellow."
And so he is.

According to Penfield, what Osler needed when he was given the gold watch was a new job—a difficult job, not a rest!

With the interest in later life issues and the emergence of studies in gerontology in the 1970s, "goal setting" emerged as a theme. The research literature at that time continued to represent a traditional male perspective, with little consideration for the different life histories of women. According to our research, the majority of women currently in their 70s and 80s had only one goal—to get a husband—and homemaking was their career. So when did they retire? When their husbands died. Which means some never did retire.

We know now that setting goals is associated with health; setting goals and *achieving* them leads to better health as well as deep satisfaction. No matter what age you are, the achievement of meaningful goals leads to greater health and psychological well-being. Remember Uncle Fred? He retired at 65 and spent a whole lot of time resting and watching TV—and died of a heart attack at the age of 66. What he needed was a purpose, a reason for getting up in the morning. When you are focused on achieving your goals, you don't have *time to kill* or *time to waste*. Remember Aunt Polly? At 94, she was determined to dance at her great-granddaughter's wedding—and she did—and died a month later.

When we have goals, we focus on what is possible. We have hope for the future.

GOAL-SETTING WORKSHOP

Compelling Reasons for Compelling Goals
Setting compelling goals is the foundation of achievement in life. Goals motivate us, they give us the energy we need to achieve success. By setting and achieving personal goals, each of us can create our own path. We become responsible for the direction of our life, in both a practical and spiritual sense. We feel like winners when we are moving toward our goals. It feels good. Most people are happiest when working toward a worthwhile goal. It is not surprising, therefore, that goal setting is basic to how we age.

> I know of no more encouraging fact than the unquestionable ability of man to elevate his life by conscious endeavor.
> —HENRY DAVID THOREAU

What follows are various approaches to goal setting. Read through all of them and pick one that you can identify with. The 10 steps work well for many people. Variations are included; pick what fits. The main point is to follow one process and expect it to work. These steps will work for you if you follow the simple instructions.

STEP 1   Set a goal you intensely desire, and go for it!
STEP 2   Write it down.
STEP 3   Write down all the advantages to achieving it.
STEP 4   Make your goal measurable.
STEP 5   Identify obstacles.
STEP 6   Identify knowledge you will need.
STEP 7   Identify people or groups that will help you reach your goal.
STEP 8   Make a plan and set a deadline.
STEP 9   Get a clear mental picture of your goal (visualize).
STEP 10 Never give up!

---

10 STEPS TO ACHIEVING YOUR GOALS

STEP 1. **Set a goal you intensely desire, and go for it!**

Your goal must be something you want for yourself. The goal cannot be something that you want for someone else. If you do not know what it is you want, what follows are some approaches and questions that will help you figure that out. The major point is to become fulfilled, to reach your potential, to become the whole and healthy person you really want to be.

Napoleon Hill is absolutely right. Your goal must be believable; you have the ability to achieve it if it is. If you want to lose weight, it is not reasonable to expect to drop from 165 pounds to 135 pounds in one month, nor is it healthy. If, however,

> There are many things in life that will catch your eye, but only a few will catch your heart...pursue those.

> What the mind can conceive and believe, it can achieve.
> —NAPOLEON HILL

your goal is to lose two pounds a week, then weight loss of thirty pounds becomes easy to achieve. Goals should stretch us but they shouldn't be so challenging that they seem impossible.

Your goal could be in any one of the following areas:

PHYSICAL   I am going to exercise more.

EMOTIONAL   I'm going to connect with three of my old friends or make new ones.

MENTAL   I'm going to learn how to play bridge or I'm going to read one history book a month.

SPIRITUAL   I'm going to learn to meditate, relax, reflect, pray.

FINANCIAL   I'm going to make a budget and live within it. I'm going to put a certain amount of money into a savings plan each year.

Here are some examples of goals that people in our mental fitness program set for themselves:

- Become a stand-up comic
- Develop a more positive attitude
- Quit smoking
- Get in touch with cousins for the first time
- Keep a daily journal
- Write a personal history for children and grandchildren
- Have more fun
- Develop a better sense of humor
- Make new friends
- Promote lifelong learning for seniors and dispel the myth of declining mental abilities with age

The following exercises are easy to do and will help you discover what you want most out of life—that is, if you don't already know. It's a curious fact that most people don't.

One straightforward way to discover what you want is to write down 10 things you want to do before you die. This is a very good place to start exploring your goals. Exercise 1: "Finding Out What You Really Want" will help you if you do it now, for it will give you a focus as you read through the book. Please give this exercise a shot. We guarantee you will like it—and you'll learn something important about yourself.

> When you pinpoint what it is you want, you're halfway there.

EXERCISE 1: **FINDING OUT WHAT YOU REALLY WANT**

Take a blank piece of paper and write at the top:

Ten things I want to do before I die.

Take about five minutes to list what they are. You don't have to think too hard about each item. After you have made the list, go back and prioritize the three most important ones. Put a "1" beside the most important, "2" beside the next most important, and "3" beside the next most important. These three items need to then be put through the 10-step goal process that begins on page 60. Commitment is the belief that motivates your persistence.

> We may affirm absolutely that nothing great in the world has ever been accomplished without passion.
>
> —GEORG HEGEL

EXERCISE 2: ANOTHER WAY TO FIND OUT WHAT YOU REALLY WANT (IF YOU DON'T ALREADY KNOW)

Answer the following questions.

1. List five values that are important to you (for example, health, love, security).

    1.

    2.

    3.

    4.

    5.

2. Take the one-minute test. List your three most important goals in life right now (for example, buy a house, create a garden, research the family tree).

    1.

    2.

    3.

3. What would you do differently if you won a million dollars?

Answers to these three questions will give you a variety of ideas to work with. Look back over what you have written. Pull out the three things that you feel excited about. These will give you a good indication as to what you really want to do or be.

FINDING YOUR PURPOSE AND PASSION

Your assignment is to pick your most important goal and put it through the 10 steps.

STEP 1: **Pick the goal that you feel most passionate about first.**
This goal has the potential to change your life forever. Remember, you have nothing to lose. You've bought the book, you've got a good start, you're on a roll—so put your brain in gear and give it a workout.

> Great minds have purposes, others have wishes.
>
> **—WASHINGTON IRVING**

STEP 2: **Write down your goal.**
This is an extremely important step. The process of writing down personal goals is what separated "the men from the boys" in the Yale study we mentioned previously. It's also what separates the women from the girls. The physical process of writing down your goal programs it into your mind. It makes it more real, more alive. In fact, until you have written down your goals, they often remain only in your dreams. Writing down goals gives you the greatest chance of achieving them. It's the foundation for success. Following are some goal examples and how to word them for success:

My goal is to do some writing. (*too vague*)
My goal is to write a romantic novel. (*specific*)

My goal is to lose weight. (*too vague*)
My goal is to lose 10 pounds. (*specific*)

My goal is to be more sociable. (*too vague*)
My goal is to make one new friend. (*specific*)

My goal is to get involved with music. (*too vague*)
My goal is to conduct an orchestra. (*specific*)

STEP 3: **Write down the advantages to achieving your goal.**
This is the step that will create the desire, the passion you need to achieve your goals. It is the step that gives you the compelling reasons you would want to put the necessary effort into achieving your goals. This is the step that tells you what the benefits are to accomplishment. Here is where you will want to list at least one dozen reasons, advantages, or benefits to achieving your goal. And once again you must write them down if you want to be successful and complete your goals. The best way to do this is in a notebook that you will keep so that you can refer back to it over the years. In my notebook, there are goals I wrote down over 10 years ago, and it gives me great satisfaction to look back over my accomplishments. It is a very healthy thing to do.

> **Goals** are not absolutely necessary to motivate us, they are **essential** to really keep us alive.
>
> —ROBERT H. SCHULLER

Let's consider some examples. First, write down your goal. We'll start with a popular one: "My goal is to lose 10 pounds." Then list the benefits:

The benefits of losing 10 pounds:
1. I'll fit into my clothes and save some money.
2. I'll look better to myself and others.
3. I'll feel better.
4. I'll have more energy.

5. I'll be more confident.
6. I'll feel more like exercising—then I'll look and feel even better.
7. I'll be able to tuck my blouse or shirt in.
8. My outlook will become more positive.
9. I won't feel so depressed.
10. I can go for that promotion in my new suit.
11. My health will improve.
12. I won't be afraid of falling on my Rollerblades.
13. My squash game will improve.
14. I'll like myself more.
15. I'll enjoy life more.
16. The quality of my entire life will improve.

All this for just 10 pounds. Wow, such a deal!

Now let's look at another goal, perhaps not as straightforward as losing weight. Let's say you have always dreamed of conducting an orchestra, but you never thought it was possible. Well, anything's possible. So let's start with the advantages of achieving this goal. Again, we'll go for at least 12 reasons. First, you write down "My goal is to conduct an orchestra." Then you list the benefits:

The benefits of conducting an orchestra are:
1. I'll subscribe to season's tickets to the symphony—for inspiration!
2. I'll get tickets with three of my friends and we'll go to dinner once a month to socialize before each concert.
3. I'll pick up my old flute that I haven't played for 25 years and see if it still works—or if I still work.
4. I'll take some lessons again—just for fun.
5. I'll research the local community orchestras and chamber music groups.

6. I'll target one I like and attend their concerts.
7. I'll study the scores for pieces at upcoming concerts—a great mental workout.
8. I'll contact a member of the orchestra through my network of family and friends, and passionately describe my dream.
9. I'll feel the thrill of standing on a podium in front of a real live orchestra.
10. I'll feel great pride in pulling this off.
11. I'll have fun sharing the experience with my family and friends.
12. I'll have renewed confidence and zest for life.

These are compelling reasons that will drive you to achieve the goal you've set.

STEP 4: **Make your goal measurable.**

Being able to measure your goals is more important than you might think. First, you need to assess your current status. For example, suppose you want to lose 30 pounds. Your goal is, therefore, to lose 30 pounds. It's an easy goal to measure—step on the scales every week and you will be able to measure your progress.

Suppose, however, your goal is to conduct an orchestra. What is your current status? *Zip.* You've never even held a baton, although you love to conduct in the privacy of your own living room when you've got Beethoven's Third Symphony blasting out of the stereo. In this case, you will know you've reached your goal—and you can reach it sooner than you think—because you'll be standing in front of a real live orchestra, baton in hand, reveling in the dream you've made come true.

We're going to use these examples throughout steps 5 to 10 to illustrate the process that you will use to achieve your goal. At this point, you have identified your goal and followed the first four steps.

STEP 5. **Identify obstacles.**

Identify any obstacles that you expect to encounter and have to over-come to reach your goal. If there are no obstacles, then it's not a goal—it's an activity. The difference bet-ween a goal and an activity is that a goal is something to achieve as a result of activities. An activity can be simply something we do with no result or purpose in mind. It may be something we have always done, or it may be something new that we do (for example, knit another afghan, go for a walk every morning).

> Obstacles are those frightful things you see when you take your eyes off your goals.
>
> —ANONYMOUS

If you write down the obstacles, you will have identified them and will then be able to incorporate how to deal with them into your plan. These barriers are important to look at—on paper. When they are written down, they don't loom as large.

In our two examples, the lists might look something like this:

Obstacles to weight loss:
1. None of my friends want to lose weight right now, and I don't like doing things on my own.
2. I can't really afford to join Weight Watchers or any other weight management club.
3. My partner loves chocolate and candy and always has it lying around.
4. I have so many pounds to lose, I'm not sure where to begin.

Obstacles to conducting an orchestra:
1. I'm embarrassed to tell my family—they'll think I'm crazy.
2. I don't know where to begin.

3. Symphony orchestras don't have time to be catering to the whim of some idiot who thinks he'd like to conduct an orchestra.

4. You have to be a world-class musician to conduct an orchestra.

Triumph is overcoming obstacles.

Now that you have identified these barriers, they can't stop you from achieving your goal. Doing the next step will motivate you to get on with it.

STEP 6: **Identify knowledge you will need.**

Any goal worth achieving requires that we learn something new. This learning pushes us to grow and develop in a healthy way. The knowledge you will need may be found in the library, by asking a specialist in a particular field, or by taking a course. So go digging!

In the weight loss example, you can find out about local support groups, perhaps even free programs, at your community center. Or you can cost out Weight Watchers and check on dates and times that would suit your schedule. It never hurts to go to the library and pick up the latest motivational book!

In the orchestra example, research the rehearsal times and find out how to get in to watch one. The school of music at the local university or a high school band will have rehearsals that you could start with. A member of the faculty or a high school music teacher could help you find out something about the symphony conductor and might even know someone who knows him or her.

Our greatest weakness lies in giving up. The most certain way to succeed is to always try just one more time.

—THOMAS EDISON

STEP 7: **Identify people or groups that will help you reach your goal.**
Write down all the people you know who will support your goals.
Pick three or four and tell them your plans and dreams. Ask each
one if he or she is willing to be your "support person"—someone you
can check in with weekly to report on your progress. These are the
people who will support you even if you have "little" progress to
report one week. If you belong to a group, ask if you may use the
group for support and take maximum advantage of the opportunity.

STEP 8: **Make a plan and set a deadline.**
How can your life go according to plan if you don't have one? The
best-laid plans of mice and men "gang aft aglay" . . . *unless you write
them down.*

In order to get to a new place, you need a road map. Mapping
out your goal as a plan—with activities, timelines, and deadlines—
is crucial if you are going to get to your
destination. Your plan needs to incorporate all the work you have done in Steps 1
to 7. Take up to three goals and prioritize
them. Then under each write the activities
you are going to engage in to accomplish
each goal. Next, beside each write a timeline and a deadline. You can revise and
rewrite the plan many times.

> I find the great thing
> in this world is not so
> much where we stand,
> as in what direction
> we are moving.
>
> —OLIVER WENDELL HOLMES

The clock of life ticks away with or without goals. Setting deadlines is essential to their achievement. In fact, goals are nothing but
dreams with a deadline.

STEP 9: **Get a clear mental picture of your goal.**
Get a clear mental picture of your goal as if you have already
achieved it. Remember Billie Jean King's words to Martina

Navratilova? At a critical point in her career, Navratilova had won all the major international tennis championships except Wimbledon, and she went to Billie Jean for coaching. Billie Jean told her to think of herself as someone who had already won Wimbledon. And, guess what?

Try out your ideas by **visualizing** them in **action.**

—DAVID SEABURY

Visualize your goal over and over until it is embedded in your mind's eye or in your mind's ear. Play it over and over and over again like a recording. Remember, you can shape your own vision of what you want to do or become by seeing yourself doing it and considering it done.

STEP 10: **Never give up!**

Back your plan with determination, persistence, and perseverance. These are the most important qualities for success. Now is the time to make a resolution to never give up. And this is where discipline comes in.

Your persistence in any endeavor is a measure of how much you believe in yourself—if you believe in yourself, you believe in your ability—if you believe in your ability, you believe in your success—if you believe in your success, what is left to stop you?

Remember Edison? Remember how he persevered despite thousands of failures? He's the one who said, "Genius is one percent inspiration and 99 percent perspiration." Or as Stephen Covey says, "Believe it and you will see it."

In Step 1, we have demonstrated the importance of setting goals, particularly when *your time is your own.* You now have a better understanding of yourself and what you value most in life. You have identified at least one personal goal—maybe even a goal that you can get passionate about, a goal that you perhaps considered to be *only in your wildest dreams.* A goal like climbing Mount Everest or conducting an orchestra. You now know all the wonderful benefits of achieving your goal and the kinds of obstacles that prevent you from achieving it. Remember, the greatest obstacle is *you* and the negative beliefs and assumptions you hold about what you are able to achieve.

The negative beliefs and assumptions about aging are the ones that are most powerful, because they are difficult to identify and difficult to change. Did your mother tell you life was going to be easy? The harder you work, the greater your sense of achievement and joy. In Step 2 we'll go beyond the limiting language you use to speak about yourself and what you are able to achieve. You will learn a new, positive language that anticipates success. Congratulations on doing the assignment—it started on page 58 with the Goal-Setting Workshop. From now on, the assignments will come at the end of each chapter.

Nothing in the world can take
the place
Of persistence.
Talent will not;
Nothing is more common than
Unsuccessful men with talent.
Genius will not;
Unrewarded genius is almost a
proverb.
Education will not;
The world is full of
educated derelicts.
Persistence and
determination
Alone are omnipotent.
—CALVIN COOLIDGE

You are never given a dream without also being given the power to make it come true. . . . You may have to work for it, however.
—RICHARD BACH

STEP 2

POWER THINKING:
GOING BEYOND *the* WORDS

The biggest change that has occurred in society in relation to aging has not been a fundamental genetic discovery that enables scientists to alter the course of aging, but a fundamentally new recognition of the power we have to grow and transform our lives as we age.

—GENE COHEN

🔔 MENTAL FITNESS WARM-UP

The congregation of a small church in England decided that the step up to the front door, which was a single stone slab, had become so worn by years of use that it would have to be replaced. Unfortunately, there were no funds available for the replacement. Then someone came up with the bright idea that the replacement could be postponed for many years.

What was the bright idea? Give this some deep thinking and try to solve it yourself—then turn to the "Clues and Answers," page 240, for the answer.

POWER THINKING

This chapter has the power to change your life. We call it "power thinking," because the process we're going to describe involves replacing negative thoughts with thoughts that provide the power and energy you need to be in charge of your mind, to accomplish your goals—or anything else you *put your mind to*.

Life is not easy for any of us. But what of that? We must have perseverance and above all confidence in ourselves. We must believe that we are gifted for something, and that this thing, at whatever cost, must be attained.

—MARIE CURIE

In the previous chapter, we explored the topic of goal setting and suggested that adults typically have negative assumptions and limited expectations about what they are capable of being and doing in their later years; these assumptions and expectations prevent them from setting ambitious goals and reaching their full potential. Those negative assumptions, the most common being "my memory is getting worse," keep people from developing new interests and enjoying life to the fullest.

When you take critical thinking to the next level—to power thinking—you empower yourself to take positive action. We have all relied to some extent on someone close to us to encourage us, someone who reflects and reinforces our positive attributes when we are hard on ourselves, someone who coaxes or coaches us on to better things. Empowering others, for example, involves believing in them, giving them the support and resources they need to develop their full potential, reinforcing and recognizing their contributions. With power thinking, you never have to wait for someone else to encourage you, because you will be able to mobilize your own personal coach whenever you need one.

You will benefit from power thinking for the rest of your life. Ultimately, when you get there—if you aren't already there—you will embrace old age as a modern miracle and a privilege. How many times have you heard someone say, "If only I had more time"? Well, you've got it now, thanks to the miracle of longevity!

Some people love the words "power" and "empowerment," some are turned off by them, and others simply never use them. We are asking you to suspend all negative thinking—if you haven't already done so—from this point forward, and be open to what you will learn and accomplish as a result of empowering thoughts.

Like Madame Curie, countless people throughout history have

made outstanding achievements in their later years. Consider the following list:

Twelve Great Achievers
These people were power thinkers. They believed they could do great things and they did—regardless of their age.

1. At 100, Grandma Moses was painting.
2. At 94, Bertrand Russell was active in the international peace movement.
3. At 93, George Bernard Shaw wrote the play *Farfetched Fables*.
4. At 91, Eamon de Valera served as president of Ireland.
5. At 91, Adolph Zukor was chairman of Paramount Pictures.
6. At 90, Pablo Picasso was producing drawings and engravings.
7. At 89, Artur Rubinstein gave one of his greatest recitals at Carnegie Hall.
8. At 89, Albert Schweitzer headed a hospital in Africa.
9. At 88, Michelangelo did architectural plans for the Church of Santa Maria degli Angeli.
10. At 88, Konrad Adenauer was chancellor of Germany.
11. At 85, Coco Chanel was the head of her own fashion design firm.
12. At 80, George Burns won an Academy Award for his performance in *The Sunshine Boys*.

In this chapter, we will review and sensitize you to some of the myths and stereotypes that are deeply embedded in the minds and hearts of people of all ages. Negative myths, internalized as negative beliefs, prevent people from getting the most out of life and giving their best back to society in important ways. Negative myths keep people from dreaming dreams and realizing them. We begin by naming the negative myths. Next, we'll explore the assumptions and beliefs for their essential merit. Then we'll give you the necessary tools to eradicate limiting beliefs and to use critical thinking skills to replace old beliefs with positive ones that reflect a more up-to-date, enlightened awareness of aging and growing older. Here's the step-by-step process we will guide you through:

1. What's new about aging
2. The time of your life
3. Identifying the negative beliefs
4. A new old age
5. Negative and positive ageism
6. Consequences of ageism
7. Current research on ageism
8. Replacing old beliefs with new beliefs
9. Critical thinking
10. Hidden assumptions
11. Power thinking
12. Challenging assumptions through critical thinking
13. Five steps to challenging your mind
14. Words for healthy aging

Let's begin with a look at what's new about aging, and why we may even look forward to it as an opportunity, a true gift of time— time to continue to grow and learn, enrich and deepen your experience of the good things in life that you value most.

I believe that we can slow and transform the aging process as we know it. I think it is possible to become more vital, energetic, and beautiful as we get older, rather than less so. So let go of the old rules and the old limitations and begin to experi-

ence day to day the wonder of a limitless life, a limitless world, a limitless universe.

—SHAKTI GAWAIN

WHAT'S NEW *About* AGING?

You have probably heard it before—and you're going to hear it again. *Thirty years have been added to the average lifespan* in the past century, and there are indications from current research that we may be able to live to 120 years in the future. The new longevity is the single most outstanding achievement of the 20th century. It presents opportunities that we are only beginning to explore as a consequence of aging populations around the world. Our goal throughout this book is to convince you that, whatever your current age, and whatever your current beliefs, you can continue to improve, keep your mind fit, and enjoy life more than you ever dreamed possible.

It's a world away from this child's view of Grandma and Grandpa living in a trailer park in Arizona:

> **THE GREATEST TEST**
>
> Do you know what the greatest test is? Do you still get excited about what you do when you get up in the morning?
>
> —DAVID HALBERSTAM

My Spring Vacation with Grandma and Grandpa

We always spend Spring Vacation with Grandma and Grandpa. They used to live up here in a big brick house but Grandpa got retarded and they moved to Arizona. They live in a park with a lot of other retarded people. They all live in tin huts. They ride tri-cycles that are too big for me. They all go to a building they call the wrecked hall but it's fixed now. They all do exercises, but not very well. They play a game with big checkers and push them around the floor with sticks. There is a swimming pool, but I guess nobody teaches them; they just stand there in the water with their hats on. My Grandma used to bake cookies but nobody cooks there. They all go to restaurants that are fast and have dis-counts. When you come into the park, there is a dollhouse with a man sitting in it. He watches them all day so they can't get out without him seeing them. I guess everybody forgets who they are because they all wear badges with their names on them. Some of them don't hear very well. They could hear better if they took the buttons out of their ears. Grandma says that Grandpa worked hard all this life to earn retardment. I wish they would come back home. I guess the man in the dollhouse won't let them out.

THE TIME *of* YOUR LIFE

It's an exciting time to be alive and growing older. In a sense, it's *in* to be *old*. Everybody wants to be a senior. Seniors are offered special reduced prices. In fact, seniors get discounts on just about every-thing, and it starts once you hit 55. People have always lied about their age, because they wanted the privileges that go along with a certain age. At 16 you get to drive a car; at 19 (or 21, depending on where you live) you get to drink beer in public; at 50 you can join a seniors' center and learn about almost anything; at 60 you can take free or low-cost courses at most universities. Seniors have it so good, people are now claiming to be *older than they really are* so they can enjoy some of the benefits.

Most people want to get all the benefits they can but don't really want to admit that they qualify for them. Is there anyone who actually aspires to be 75 or 85 or 95? It's a conundrum. Consider the following:

Did you realize . . .

- If you're less than 10 years old, you're so excited about aging that you think in fractions. How old are you? "I'm four and a half" . . . You're never 36 and a half . . . you're four and a half going on five!
- That's the key. You get into your teens—now they can't hold you back. You jump to the next number. How old are? "I'm gonna be 16."
- And then something truly momentous happens . . . you become 21. Even the words sound like a ceremony . . . you *become* 21 . . .
- You *become* 21, you turn 30, then you're *pushing* 40 . . . you *reach* 50 . . . then you *make it* to 60 . . . Whew! I didn't think I'd make it. And then you build up so much speed you *hit* 70! After that, it is a day-by-day thing. After that, you *hit* Wednesday . . .
- You get into your 80s, you *hit* lunch. My grandmother won't even buy green bananas . . . "Well, it's an investment you know, and maybe a bad one."
- And it doesn't end there . . . into the 90s you start going backwards . . . I was *just* 92.
- Then a strange thing happens. If you make it over 100, you become a little kid again . . . "I'm 100 and a half!"

IDENTIFYING *the* NEGATIVE BELIEFS

Deep down, most people are terrified of aging. What are the myths and images of old age that prevent people from being the best they can be right to the end? Let's examine a recent newspaper article to identify the stereotypes and the less obvious negative beliefs that support the stereotypes. Myths, by definition, are common beliefs that are simply not true. What are the myths or assumptions in the following article? What are the unstated negative beliefs that feed on them? What's the evidence that they are not true?

I took my children to Disney World but they missed the parade. The place was swamped with old people. All my kids saw were plaid shorts and varicose veins. If you've never been to Florida, prepare for the world's premier collection of impaired drivers. Everywhere you look, gnarled old ladies or withered walnut-colored men peer over steering wheels. . . . I'm sick of old people. I'm tired of their gigantic wrap-around glasses. Mostly, I'm tired of subsidizing a mushrooming class of deadbeats. Over the last 15 years, income for seniors has risen at a faster rate than any other age group. Men who are 65 or older generate an average of 46% of their income from public pension and benefits. That, friends, is a welfare bum. . . . The aged are our most militant deadbeats and they want to make sure nobody nudges them from their prime spot on the public trough. . . . When you hear an old person moaning over discounted coffee about the deficit or the bums on welfare, tell them they can make a worthwhile contribution . . . just die already. . . . I say freeze 'em when they hit 75. . . . Difficult times, the elderly constantly tell us, require difficult decisions. Freeze them. Freeze them now while we still can.

What do you think? Is this for real? Or is the author just having fun? Where does he get these images? Before you respond to the article, let's consider a brief history of old age and "ageism"—a theme that is central to the field of gerontology. "Ageism" is, in short, the manifestation through language of negative beliefs and attitudes about old people. We're going to survey the last 40 years for an understanding of ageism, and consider whether society is making progress in overcoming the myths and stereotypes. Are we really entering a new age where old age can be embraced?

Before we get back to what's new about aging and how we can integrate that new reality into our lives as aging people in an aging world, we are going to give you a greater appreciation for history. A historical perspective sheds new light on the present . . . and hope for the future.

Our concept of age and what it means to be old is constantly changing. To put you in a historical frame of mind, we'd like you to consider some of the changes that have occurred since 1918:

- The average life expectancy in North America was 47.
- Only 14 percent of the homes in North America had a bathtub. Only 8 percent of the homes had a telephone.
- The maximum speed limit in most cities was 10 miles per hour.
- The tallest structure in the world was the Eiffel Tower.
- More than 95 percent of all births in North America took place at home.
- Sugar cost four cents a pound. Eggs were fourteen cents a dozen. Coffee cost fifteen cents a pound.
- Most women washed their hair only once a month.
- The five leading causes of death in North America were
  1. Pneumonia and influenza
  2. Tuberculosis
  3. Diarrhea
  4. Heart disease
  5. Stroke
- Drive-by shootings—in which teenage boys galloped down the street on horses and started randomly shooting at houses, carriages, or anything else that caught their fancy—were an ongoing problem in Denver and other cities in the west.

- Plutonium, insulin, and antibiotics hadn't been discovered yet. Scotch tape, crossword puzzles, canned beer, and iced tea hadn't been invented.
- There was no Mother's Day or Father's Day.
- One in ten North American adults couldn't read or write. Only 6 percent of all Americans had graduated from high school.
- Some medical authorities warned that professional seamstresses were apt to become sexually aroused by the steady rhythm of the sewing machine's foot pedal. They recommended slipping bromide—which was thought to diminish sexual desire—into their drinking water.
- Marijuana, heroin, and morphine were all available over the counter at corner drugstores. According to one pharmacist, "Heroin clears the complexion, gives buoyancy to the mind, regulates the stomach and the bowels, and is, in fact, a perfect guardian of health."
- Coca-Cola contained cocaine instead of caffeine.

The time has come to review and renew the meaning of old age. During the 20th century, medical science has succeeded in extending the human life span by more than 20 years, but we really don't have a legitimate social role for those added 20 or 30 years. In the 1960s and 1970s, demographers ominously predicted the graying of America. Viewing older people generally as passive, dependent, non-contributing members of society, they warned of the inevitable increase in the burden to society of caring for catastrophic numbers of elderly people. During those two decades, gerontology was developed and firmly established as a science and a profession.

Today, the graying of populations in developing countries around the world is a fact of life. With a membership of 33 million people, the American Association of Retired People (AARP) is the second largest voluntary organization in the United States. Organizations representing older people are growing throughout the world. The numbers aren't surprising, but no one anticipated the emerging face of old age.

While the numbers were growing, a second and much quieter revolution was taking place. The face of old age was changing, and a new breed of *Homo sapiens* was emerging. Those who got to know them found that older people were much more vital and interesting than they'd ever anticipated. Those who listened to their life stories marveled at their courage, their creativity, their passion, their deep understanding of human nature and the meaning of life. Older people who seemed "ordinary," neither wealthy nor elite, seemed somehow exceptional and extraordinary. Like the woman who climbed Mount Everest in her 80s. The African-American student from Louisiana who learned to read at 94. The First Nations student from the Pacific Northwest who graduated from high school at 94. The woman who became blind in her 80s, took six months to learn a keyboard by touch, and published her first book at 92—with four more in the works. The woman in her 80s who was raped and beaten in her apartment, moved to a nursing home with tight security, and then moved on to campaign for public safety for seniors.

Despite these changes, myths and assumptions about old age linger, left over from a reality that no longer exists. Blinded by ageist beliefs, many people don't recognize the wisdom and strength of people who are older, and so fail to nurture the infinite possibilities within each of us. No wonder so many retired people talk about feeling "invisible"—no one sees them as individuals, only as older people.

Not only do the ageist stereotypes die hard, they serve as self-fulfilling prophecies for the majority of older people. People learn how to grow old by watching other people grow old, severely limiting the possibilities for growth and productivity. The challenge is to reconstruct the meaning of old age, to view the aging of society as the unprecedented triumph that it is, and to envision possibilities for growth and productivity unknown in human history. It's time to "give your head a shake and get an attitude."

A NEW OLD AGE

The subject of old age has always been fraught with ambivalence. Most people have compassion for old people, but shrink from the image of an aging self. Everyone loves "Grandma," but few aspire to be like her. Ageism is insidious in many societies, subtle and pervasive, affecting not just senior citizens but all members of society. Yet rarely is it recognized and addressed. Getting beyond simple negative or positive stereotypes requires a fundamental shift from viewing older people as "the problem," to viewing them as most capable of helping younger generations to understand the *real* problems, and work together to develop creative solutions.

Grandma's Glasses

A little boy said to a playmate, "When I get older I want to wear glasses just like Grandma wears. She must have a special kind because she can see so much more than most people. She can see how to fix a lot of things to have fun with, and she can see when I try to do something even if I don't do it right. She can see when I am sad and she can see what to do to make me feel better. I asked her one day how she sees so good, and she said it was the way she learned to look at things as she got older. When I get older I want a pair of glasses just like Grandma's so I can see good too."

—From *The War Cry*

How shall we best describe the majority of older people today? Older people are generally perceived as healthier, better-educated, and richer. Furthermore, this growing population of people who just happen to be older will require opportunities for higher education and involvement in volunteer and/or work roles once family responsibilities diminish. This group generally has the money and education to take care of its own needs, and because many do not want to grow old, they will seek high-tech options to help them stay young forever. Money is no problem—the real problem is growing old.

What does it mean to be "old" in a society that celebrates youth? Consider the following:

"Old" is when your sweetie says, "Let's go upstairs and make love," and you answer, "Honey, I can't do both!"

"Old" is when a sexy babe catches your fancy and your pacemaker opens the garage door.

"Old" is when you don't care where your spouse goes, just as long as you don't have to go along.

"Old" is when you are cautioned to slow down by the doctor instead of by the police.

"Old" is when "getting lucky" means finding your car in the parking lot.

"Old" is when an "all-nighter" means not getting up to pee!

NEGATIVE *and* POSITIVE AGEISM

Just as society is beginning to recognize that older people have much to contribute, we must be aware that "positive ageism" is as limiting as the negative attitudes. A study by John Bell, formerly a researcher based at the City University of New York, explored images of the elderly on television as powerful, affluent, physically and socially active, smart, admired by others, sexually attractive but not sexually active, and not dealing with real problems. His findings are contrasted with the characterizations of older adults prior to the 1980s as rarely smart, attractive, active, or sexy.

This kind of tabloid thinking suggests all old people are well off, in good health, and able to take care of themselves. Previously this pie-in-the-sky attitude was ignored, but positive ageism is becoming as great a problem as negative ageism, because it leads to a number of negative consequences for individuals and for society.

CONSEQUENCES *of* AGEISM

Societies around the world will continue to suffer the consequences of both negative and positive ageism until every person has legitimate opportunities for personal development and productive engagement well beyond the traditional age of retirement. Personal costs are loss of self-esteem, loss of function, loss of self-confidence, and physical and mental decline. These are exacerbated by the current economic strains on older people in the form of government budget cuts and the public focus on the cost of health care and other benefits for the elderly. The greatest economic cost, however, is seldom mentioned: we are wasting the productive and creative abilities of millions of older people who retire because they are 65.

Ageism is insidious in many societies, subtle and pervasive, affecting not just senior citizens but all members of society. Yet rarely is it recognized and addressed. Getting beyond simple negative or positive stereotypes requires a fundamental shift from viewing older people as "the problem" to viewing them as capable of helping younger generations to understand the real problems and to develop creative solutions.

The primary challenge is to develop a legitimate social purpose for those added 20 or 30 years. That is the challenge for all of us, collectively, as a society. And it is the challenge for each and every one of us who share the possibility of living to a very old age. Do you have a mission, role, or goal for the next 10, 20, or 30 years that gives your life meaning? If not, how will you develop a role for yourself?

Given that the wealthiest people are over 50, the cohort of older adults would seem to have the means and resources to cope with their own aging. The hidden assumption behind a growing political agenda in many countries around the world is that this same group will also assume society's burden of caring, economically and in kind, for the even more dramatically growing numbers of frail elderly people. Corporate America's new image of aging has resulted in positive stereotyping: healthy, active older people spend their time playing golf, going on luxury cruises, enjoying fine restaurants. Do we really imagine that they are prepared to take care of others who are not so fortunate? Furthermore—and shattering the tabloid image altogether—do we believe that older people really want to spend the rest of their lives in self-indulgent pursuits?

CURRENT RESEARCH *on* AGEISM

Toward the end of the 20th century, we find more encouraging research that suggests we are making progress; certainly, we have a greater understanding and heightened awareness of the issues. Many people believe that older women suffer more from ageism than men do because it is compounded by sexism—in other words, appearance is more important to women than men. One study by

Patricia Sharpe from the University of Texas at Austin entitled "Older Women and Health Services: Moving from Ageism Toward Empowerment" suggests ageism and sexism in health services and research affect the quality of care, patient–provider interaction, patient self-perceptions, and the planning of health education programs for older women. Prevailing research is focused on disease processes and neglects the subjective experience of older women. Changes at the organizational, community, and individual levels that promote the autonomy and empowerment of older women are discussed.

> There are three classes into which all the women past seventy years of age I have ever known were divided: that dear old soul; that old woman; that old witch.
>
> —SAMUEL TAYLOR COLERIDGE

A study by Amanda Smith-Barusch from the University of Utah examined the extent to which low-income older women describe themselves in negative terms, and the strategies they use to preserve their self-esteem. The study reveals that, instead of considering themselves "old" or "poor," they defined themselves as "fortunate" or "blessed." The author suggests that the ability to see oneself as fortunate may be a significant component of successful aging. In other words, they had a positive mental attitude (see Step 4).

Amanda Smith-Barusch explored literature on "the crone" from a feminist perspective. Crones, hags, and witches have negative connotations in modern Western society that feed negative stereotypes of the "old woman." Feminist scholars in particular have expressed the need to produce valued images of the old woman's body, to reclaim the crone in cultural representations where old women have been largely effaced. Remember the phrase, getting together with "old cronies"? That phrase is used in a non-pejorative sense to refer to long-time friends, whether male or female. More recently, the tradition of "croning" has been resurrected and practiced as a positive rite of passage for women turning 60 years of age.

Kimberly Sieber, a researcher with a life-span perspective, focused on self-concept. A total of 210 men and women from younger, middle-aged, and older age groups were compared on measures of self-esteem and self-concept with respect to role (e.g., self as mother, self as scholar, self as grandfather). There were no age group or sex differences in self-esteem; however, compared to younger adults, older adults expressed stronger beliefs in their goodness and virtue, as well as their ability to effectively complete tasks. In general, for men, self-esteem and self-concept are associated with achievement whereas self-esteem for women is more often associated with the social relations. Finally, this study explored the relationships between self-concept and common life changes, such as reduced income and poor health, and other losses, such as death of a spouse, divorce, and being retired. In general, loss of income, health, spouse, or employment was different for each individual, suggesting that one's self-concept can be altered in response to life changes.

Irek Celejewski and Karen Dion examined self-perceptions of old and young adults using questionnaires from 101 college students, aged 18 to 29, and 68 older adults, aged 61 to 94. As expected, older adults evaluated elderly persons more favorably than younger adults. In addition, older adults' self-evaluations and those of young adults asked to imagine themselves as elderly were more positive than the ratings made by respondents who evaluated an unfamiliar older adult.

In a study of corporate America's tabloid view of aging from a male perspective, K.E. McHugh from the University of Arizona examines and critiques the concept of the "ageless self" and highlights expression as a potential societal script in "successful aging," focusing on the activities of the Arizona Office of Senior Living (OSL) and public/private efforts to promote Arizona as an idyllic haven for active, affluent older adults. The concept of the ageless self plays nicely into the prolongation of midlife. Nowhere is the image of the ageless self more apparent (and transparent) than in Sun Belt retirement communities where active, affluent older adults live in a blissful and perpetual state of mature adulthood. The concept of age-less self—intended as a corrective to negative stereotypes of old age—is itself ageist in that it adulates continuity and coherence as reflected in views of middle age and conveys little about change and what it means to grow old. In addition, it reflects deeply embedded societal attitudes and cultural values invested in the image of hand-some, healthy, comfortable, middle-class older adults busily filling sun-filled days.

Is this unique to North America? What about other countries and cultures? We tend to assume that other cultures respect their elders. In Europe, Peter Oberg from the University of Minnesota explored the body image among men and women over the life course, based on a survey of 2,002 Swedes, aged 20 to 85. Compared to men, women value appearance more and are more worried about bodily changes as they grow older; but the majority are content with their bodies. One interpretation is that negative images in the media create worries about age-related changes, but these worries do not correspond to actual experience.

Becca Levy from Yale University compared Japanese, American, and Chinese images of aging. She looked at the inner self of the Japanese as a defense against negative stereotypes of aging. The study showed that the Japanese elderly express more negative atti-tudes toward old people in general, but more positive self-concepts than elders in both the People's Republic of China and the United States. Questionnaire data from urban residents of all three countries (total = 150, aged 15 to 90) support this pattern. It is suggested that an unusual dynamic of aging and self-identity can be found in Japan, which sheds light on the role of the self in accepting or rejecting societal stereotypes about aging.

In Australia, Victor Minichiello and colleagues from the University of New England conducted an in-depth study of older adults (aged 65 to 89) living in urban and rural settings; they examined perceptions and consequences of ageism. Participants responded to questions about (a) the meaning of the word "ageism," (b) what constitutes ageism, (c) their experiences of ageism, (d) their perceptions of social attitudes toward older people, and (e) their personal views and experiences of becoming older. While the term "ageism" was neither understood nor used by many of the participants, they did report negative experiences in "being seen as old" and "being treated as old."

Active aging was viewed as a positive way of presenting and interpreting oneself as separate from the "old" group. Participants recognized that older people as a group experience negative treatment with regard to poor access to transportation and housing, low incomes, forced retirement, and inadequate nursing home care. While few had experienced overt ageism, their everyday interactions involved some negative treatment and occasional positive "sageism" (such as patronizing attitudes, false deference). Several participants noted that other people tend to "keep watch," monitoring older adults for signs of "incipient oldness." Health professionals were a major source of ageist treatment. Findings suggest that some older adults limit their lives by accommodating ageism, while others actively create new images of aging for themselves and those who will be old in the future.

The most interesting research for us, because of its direct application to mental abilities, was Becca Levy's study of the effect of ageism on mental fitness. This research demonstrates that subliminally activated stereotypes can alter judgments about oneself and can change mental ability. In the first study, an intervention that activated positive stereotypes of aging without the participants' awareness improved memory performance, memory self-efficacy, and views of aging in older individuals. In contrast, an intervention that activated negative stereotypes and aging tended to worsen memory performance, memory self-efficacy, and views of aging in older participants.

A second study demonstrated that for the strong effects to emerge from the shifting stereotypes, the stereotypes must be important to the individual's self-image. Young people randomly assigned to the same conditions as the older participants in the first study did not exhibit any of the significant interactions that emerged among the old participants. This research highlights the potential for memory improvement in older individuals when the negative stereotypes of aging are shifted to more positive stereotypes. In fact, all we have to do is change the ageist stereotypes to positive, and we can expect a positive result. Now, that's exciting news!

Becca Levy's most recent study explores how thoughts, feelings, and behaviors toward elderly people operate without conscious awareness within every person who has internalized the age stereotypes of their culture. She refers to ageism as "the enemy within" because it operates without awareness and has a powerful effect on older adults themselves in many areas of their lives. For example, "aging self-stereotypes can influence older individuals' cardiovascular function without their awareness."

Because stereotypes are so prevalent and so destructive in North American society, Erdman Palmore from Duke University has developed a new "Ageism Survey" that is intended to make people more aware of the many forms of ageism that they and others may be perpetrating and experiencing. Have you experienced any of the following?

The Ageism Survey
1. I was told a joke that pokes fun at older people.
2. I was sent a birthday card that pokes fun at old people.
3. I was ignored or not taken seriously because of my age.
4. I was called an insulting name related to my age.
5. I was patronized or "talked down to" because of my age.
6. I was refused rental housing because of my age.
7. I had difficulty getting a loan because of my age.
8. I was denied a position of leadership because of my age.
9. I was rejected as unattractive because of my age.
10. I was treated with less dignity and respect because of my age.
11. A waiter or waitress ignored me because of my age.
12. A doctor or nurse assumed my ailments were caused by my age.
13. I was denied medical treatment because of my age.
14. I was denied employment because of my age.
15. I was denied promotion because of my age.
16. Someone assumed that I could not hear well because of my age.
17. Someone assumed I could not understand because of my age.
18. Someone told me, "You're too old for that."
19. I was victimized by a criminal because of my age.

Only negative forms of ageism are included in this survey in order to keep it simple. Palmore's preliminary findings show (1) little difference between men and women in the number of items reported and (2) people with less education experience more ageism than those with more education.

Our goal is to sensitize you to every experience of ageism in your life and to give you the tools to eradicate every last experience you ever had or will have in the future that may be ageist. Ultimately, we intend to renew and restore a positive image of aging and respect for older people around the world.

We are making some progress in overcoming negative attitudes and beliefs that have been with us for years. Certainly, many writers now refer to the terrible waste of natural resources when older people who are healthy and able and active are restricted from participating fully in society. People are beginning to apply the results of the new brain research and are reporting strong, positive results.

What are the current facts, the positive results that we can use to challenge those old, negative beliefs and stereotypes? Burn the following facts on aging into your brain and you are on your way to a richer, more successful, more fulfilling time of your life.

New Facts of Aging

1. People grow up and grow old with hidden limiting beliefs about aging based on a reality that no longer exists.
2. The average life span is 80 years and climbing.
3. Old age is a gift of time.
4. Mental decline with age is not inevitable.
5. Any mental decline with normal aging is either "atrophy" or disease.
6. Mental decline from disuse can be reversed with a short training program.
7. With mental stimulation, the brain can continue to grow new branches into very old age.
8. In addition to growing new dendrites or branches, we can actually grow new brain cells.
9. Playing bridge or other card games has a positive effect on the immune system.

10. Anxiety about memory loss is a major cause of memory loss. Reducing anxiety alone results in improved memory.

11. Learning something new and unfamiliar—a new language, a new subject, playing an instrument—is possible and beneficial at any age.

12. There are no limits to what we can learn, be, and do at any age, *if we are prepared to do serious, hard work.*

13. The world is in desperate need of the wisdom of its elders.

14. Younger people suffer the most from ageism.

15. Learning is possible at every age.

Think back over the past 20 or 30 or even 50 years. Add to the list all the things people told you you couldn't or shouldn't do—and yet you went ahead and did them. Then read your list over . . . and over . . . and over . . . and keep it handy as we move on to replace all the old assumptions that have been holding you back.

REPLACING OLD BELIEFS *with* NEW BELIEFS

We are going to try to make a clean sweep of things in the remaining pages of this chapter. We are going to clear out the old research, old knowledge, old beliefs, and old assumptions that no longer apply to the world of today and tomorrow, and we are going to replace them with new knowledge, new beliefs, and new language. Replacing them will create greater health, greater achievement, a more positive attitude, and more enjoyment in life.

Gerontologists in the past have typically believed that the way to change attitudes was simply to offer new knowledge through university courses. Certainly, knowledge is the basis for what we believe to be true. But few of the early studies on ageism and attitude change showed a positive effect through simple knowledge acquisition. Otherwise, we could just give people the facts. That's not enough. That's where critical thinking comes into the picture.

CRITICAL THINKING

The early research on critical thinking defined it as clear, logical analysis of a problem or challenge. Scientists, for example, had to be critical thinkers. However, critical thinking as it has been developed and practiced within the adult education movement, associated with the work of Jack Mezirow and Stephen Brookfield at Columbia University, is a more practical and productive activity.

> Failures are divided into two classes: Those who thought and never did, And those who did and never thought.
>
> —JOHN CHARLES SALAK

Critical thinking as a tool has been adopted and adapted for just about every discipline and age group. There is "Critical Thinking for Teachers," "Critical Thinking for Children," "Critical Thinking for English Literature," "Critical Thinking for the Creative Arts." And now there is critical thinking for a specific topic—for people who are aging in an aging world. Being a critical thinker is part of what it means to be a developing person, and fostering critical thinking is essential to creating and maintaining a healthy aging society. Critical thinking empowers us to continually question the hidden assumptions that restrict and inhibit us from achieving our potential as human beings.

HIDDEN ASSUMPTIONS

Now it's time to test your assumptions. Refer to the picture below and respond to each of the following statements by writing "true" or "false" or "I don't know" at the end of the statement.

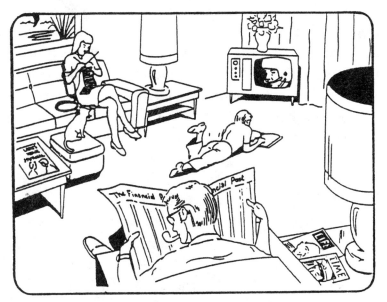

The Smith Family

1. There are three people in the room. _____
2. The Smith family owns a TV set. _____
3. There is a football game on TV. _____
4. Bobby Smith is doing his homework while watching TV. _____
5. Mrs. Smith is knitting. _____
6. The Smiths have a pet cat. _____
7. The Smiths subscribe to *Time, Life,* and *Ladies' Home Journal.* _____
8. This picture shows the family together in the evening. _____

Most people will answer yes or no to the statements. But when you stop to think about it, you may have made a number of assumptions. In statement 1, we see three people in the picture; there may be two others in the room standing behind the artist. In statement 2, there is a TV set in the room. It could be rented. They could be at Grandma's. Go back through each statement and you will begin to see that for each statement "I don't know" is the correct response. This exercise illustrates how much we operate on assumptions. We all do, because we often have to. We can't know everything. We need to be aware of assumptions, however, particularly ones that hinder us.

That's where power thinking comes into the picture.

POWER THINKING

Power thinking goes beyond critical thinking—it's critical thinking with value added. And the added value is a way of thinking that gives you the power you need to change your life. Whereas critical thinking skills are used to identify inaccurate assumptions and replace them with more accurate statements about what is true, power thinking goes beyond to identify the belief systems behind the assumptions, to *replace* the belief systems and actually change the language we use so that our speech serves us well.

Thinking and speaking in new ways help us to develop, grow, create, and maintain all aspects of health. We have greater self-esteem; we feel more confident; we challenge ageist stereotypes wherever and whenever they occur; we speak confidently and people listen in a different way to what we have to say.

Power thinkers . . .

- are flexible and open to new ideas and points of view.
- are sensitive to language and particularly aware of "limiting language."
- are positive and optimistic in their approach to life and learning.
- speak their minds whenever they are confronted with limiting language and negative attitudes.
- seek a deeper understanding of issues of aging and value old age for the opportunities and challenges it presents.
- challenge negative stereotypes of aging reflected in the media.
- take every opportunity to educate others (their peers, family and friends, and people of all ages) about the importance of learning and the particular value of mental fitness all through life.

CHALLENGING ASSUMPTIONS *Through* CRITICAL THINKING

In his book *Developing Critical Thinkers*, Stephen Brookfield lays out a method of critical thinking that is designed to challenge the beliefs and assumptions we hold that may be either erroneous or no longer useful. First, he provides insights into assumptions and how we acquire them:

> *Assumptions are the seemingly self-evident rules about reality that we use to help us seek explanations, make judgments, or decide on various actions. They are the unquestioned givens that, to us, have the status of self-evident truths. People cannot reach adulthood without bringing with them frameworks of understanding and sets of assumptions that under-gird their decisions, judgments, and actions. These assumptions influence how we understand cause-and-effect relationships (for example, seeing crime as*

the result of poverty as opposed to laziness). They inform our criteria regarding what is good behavior in others (for example, showing concern for others' misfortunes, ignoring conventional mores, ruthlessly pursuing self-interest). Assumptions help construct our understanding of what we judge to be "human nature." They fundamentally influence how we conceive of the duties and obligations that determine what is seen as appropriate conduct in personal relationships. Finally, they shape how we view the political world. They help us decide what rights we think individual citizens have, and what obligations governments may legitimately expect from us.

Critical thinking is a productive and positive activity. People who think critically are fully engaged in life, they work at their personal development, they are self-confident, they appreciate creativity, are innovative, and live as though life is full of possibilities both in the here and now and in the future. These are characteristics that we all want.

Critical thinking is a process that involves continually questioning our assumptions. It's a never-ending thought process that enables us to challenge any claims to universal truth or certainty. It is a dynamic process. Just as we used to imagine the world was flat and with total certainty we believed we could "walk off the face of the world"—but no one ever got to the edge and today we argue with total certainty that the world is round.

Critical thinking varies with every person and every situation. For some, their thinking is evident in their writing; for others, it is evident in their actions. Critical thinking is also triggered by happy or fulfilling events like success at work. When this happens, we begin to look at our actions and ideas in new ways, from a new perspective, and realize that new possibilities lie within us.

Emotions are central to the critical thinking process. When we ask ourselves about our values, ideas, and behaviors, this usually triggers great emotion. Challenging old beliefs, for instance, can cause people to feel confused and resentful as they feel they are being criticized. Relief and exhilaration are felt as people break through their old thought patterns to new ways of looking at long-held assumptions. As we realize that we have the power to change aspects of our lives, we become excited and experience a new sense of potential and freedom.

There are two main reasons why it is in your best interest to explore your assumptions. First, it creates a sense of new possibility. And second, you can reinvent a healthier way to live. In our work with older adults, critical thinking skills are an effective technique to challenge the assumptions we have about aging that limit the options we have for a healthy old age. These thinking skills are also effective in changing negative beliefs to positive beliefs that support limitless possibilities for growth and development in later life. The challenge is to create a new perspective of old age by changing our belief systems based on new research in aging that is more hopeful and optimistic.

Believe nothing on the faith of traditions, even though they have been held in honor for many generations, and in diverse places. Do not believe a thing because many speak of it. Do not believe on the faith of the sages of the past. Do not believe what you have imagined, persuading yourself that a god inspires you. Believe nothing on the sole authority of your masters or priests. After examination, believe what you yourself have tested and found to be reasonable, and confirm your conduct thereto.

—GAUTAMA BUDDHA

> One does not "find oneself" by pursuing one's self, but on the contrary be pursuing something else and learning through discipline or routine . . . who one is and wants to be.
>
> —MAY SARTON

Assumptions underlie our actions—actions and decisions spring from our assumptions. We need to have informed beliefs, not beliefs that come from old ways of thinking and doing. Critical thinking challenges these old thought patterns. Creating new thoughts can fuel long-lasting vitality. Think about it—what beliefs do you hold about aging, old age, mental function, memory, learning? These are good questions to reflect upon. Most people would say, "My mental function will decline, my memory is already not what it used to be, and I have trouble concentrating when I learn anything new." There is no question that's a gloomy picture, and unfortunately most people really believe it.

We look at our assumptions in a trauma or during a health crisis or death of a loved one, but real critical thinking should happen before a crisis. Comfortably held beliefs are not easy to let go of. We need to be open to change and open to stretching our minds. We all have assumptions and many previously dearly held beliefs may not be accurate or helpful to you. Consider the following story from *Awaken the Giant Within* by Anthony Robbins.

The Four-Minute Mile

Do you know the story of the four-minute mile? For thousands of years, people held the belief that it was impossible for a human being to run the mile in less than four minutes. But in 1954, Roger Bannister broke this imposing belief barrier. He got himself to achieve the "impossible" not merely by physical practice but by constantly rehearsing the event in his mind, breaking through the

*four-minute barrier so many times with so much emotional inten-
sity that he created vivid references that became an unquestioned
command to his nervous system to produce the result. Many people
don't realize, though, that the greatest aspect of his breakthrough
was what it did for others. In the whole history of the human race
no one had ever been able to break a four-minute mile, yet within
one year of Roger's breaking the barrier, 37 other runners also broke
it. His experience provided them with references strong enough to
create a sense of certainty that they, too, could "do the impossible."
And the year after that, 300 other runners did the same thing!*

New and better beliefs are the ones that allow the best use of your
strength and abilities and talents. New beliefs may make you mentally fitter and help improve your memory, as we will demonstrate.
What follows is a simple but very effective step-by-step process for
changing your assumptions and beliefs about aging or anything
else that is negative or limiting.

FIVE STEPS *to* CHALLENGING YOUR MIND

1. Become aware of assumptions. After completing the Smith
   family exercise and reading to this point, you are now aware of
   the assumptions that all of us make.
2. Identify the negative language that limits your thinking. In other
   words, name the assumption. For example: "I forget where I put
   things. . . . I am always forgetting where I put my keys."
3. Identify the limiting belief that underlies the negative language.
   For example, with reference to the negative language in 2, the
   limiting belief is "I believe that my mental ability is going to
   decline as I get older."

4. Challenge your limiting beliefs by asking yourself if they are true. Assessing their validity casts doubt on these beliefs—just what you want to do. You don't always forget your keys, and there is a simple strategy that will help you always remember where you put them (see Step 5 on Learning and Memory). Current research no longer supports this outdated thinking. Having this belief does not serve you in any way. It is self-defeating. And, besides, your mental ability will improve with age, not decline, if you incorporate the suggestions and strategies in this book.

5. Learn how to change them. There are a number of strategies to help you destroy the beliefs that limit you and no longer serve you in a positive way. Try them all and pick one or two that work for you. Question or doubt the old belief. It may seem that I forget my keys a lot and perhaps I do. However, it may be that I am using aging and poor memory as an excuse for being lazy and forgetful. In fact, I probably forgot things even more when I was young. Here are some strategies for dealing with old beliefs:

   - *Ridicule them.* Keys don't have feet. They don't get up and move on their own. They don't fly either. I can learn a strategy to remember where I put them. My brain is as good as when I was five. In fact, it's better.

   - *Link them to pain.* This old belief about always forgetting where I put things is causing me tremendous stress and worry. Sometimes when I can't find something I get so flustered and angry that it feels like my heart is going to jump out of my chest.

   - *Erase them.* It might sound silly, but it works. Carry an eraser around with you. When you hear yourself using negative language, take out your eraser and erase that language from your mind. We use this technique in our mental fitness classes. You'll be amazed at how it raises your awareness—and clears your mind of garbage.

- *Criticize them.* You're a useless belief. You are not helping me in any way. I am going to get rid of you once and for all.
- *Create an argument.* Replace the old belief with a new one, using the language of possibility. As we age our memories can actually improve. Now research is demonstrating that if we stimulate and challenge the brain, our mental abilities will serve us until we die.

Power Thinking in Action

Our beliefs have tremendous power, more power than most of us realize. For example, your beliefs can determine the impact that drugs have on your body. Most people know of the strong effects of a placebo—a sugar pill given to a patient in place of a drug. Consider the groundbreaking experiment in which 100 medical students were asked to participate in testing two new drugs: one was described as a super-stimulant in a red capsule, the other as a super-tranquilizer in a blue capsule. Unbeknownst to the students, the contents of the capsules had been switched: the red capsule was actually a barbiturate, and the blue capsule was actually an amphetamine. Yet half the students developed physical reactions that went along with their expectations—exactly the opposite of the chemical reaction the drugs should

Live with **intention**:

Walk to the edge,

Listen hard,

Play with abandon,

Laugh,

Choose with **no regret**,

Continue to learn,

Appreciate your friends,

Do what **you love!**

Live as if this is all there is!

have produced in their bodies! These students were not just given placebos, they were given actual drugs. But their beliefs overrode the chemical impact of the drug on their bodies.

What about negative thinking? If positive thinking can make you well, can negative thinking make you sick? Let's consider this chain of events: a patient on a cardiac ward in a Catholic hospital takes a turn for the worse and is about to die. His doctor calls a priest to administer last rites. He performs the ritual on the not-so-sick patient in the next bed, who dies within 15 minutes.

This true story, told by Herbert Spiegel, M.D., a New York City psychiatrist, is a dramatic example of how negative beliefs—whether expressed by yourself or someone else—can have a frightening impact on health. Named the "nocebo effect," the opposite of the placebo effect (the idea that positive thinking can improve health), this phenomenon has traditionally explained everything from voodoo death to the stories of medical students who develop the illnesses they study.

Now negative thinking is being held responsible for modern maladies. According to Herbert Benson, M.D., an associate professor at Harvard Medical School, a staggering 60 to 90 percent of common medical conditions can be exacerbated by the nocebo effect: chest pain, headache, asthma—all conditions for which there may not be a specific cause, such as a type of bacteria or virus. These ailments can be influenced by stress, which, in turn, may be influenced by our thoughts.

Although scientists can't pinpoint how negative thoughts may contribute to illness, brain research is unveiling intriguing possibilities. For instance, areas of the brain where the most basic of human responses—fear, for example—are expressed are connected to places in the brain that directly affect key organs, such as the heart. So if a person is afraid, she could trigger life-threatening irregular heartbeats. Does this mean that if you fear you'll develop breast cancer, you will? Not if you neutralize your fear with facts. Says Dr. Spiegel, "Irrational fear is most harmful."

Emotions affect the physical body. The language we use and the thoughts they convey influence the chemistry of the body. Language is probably one of the most powerful drugs known to man. The words we hear and the words we choose have a significant effect on our minds and our bodies. Many of us choose our words unconsciously, and these very words describe our thoughts. Strong words give us strength, weak words lessen our strength. Language can reinforce limiting beliefs; therefore, choose strong, healthy words that will ensure strong, healthy beliefs.

> Think **excitement,** talk excitement, act out excitement and you are bound to become an **excited person.** Life will take on a **new zest,** deeper interest, and **greater meaning.**
>
> —NORMAN VINCENT PEALE

How often have we said, while waiting for an appointment, "I'm *killing time*"? Some wise person said, "Killing time murders opportunities," and it's true if you think about it. This is a good example of what we call "limiting language." Because the language prevents us from taking advantage of the time. Better if we said, "I have a gift of time"—even though the waiting can be annoying. If we have to wait anyway, we can turn it into a healthy experience, rather than an unhealthy waste of time.

WORDS *for* HEALTHY AGING

LIMITING LANGUAGE	THE LANGUAGE OF POSSIBILITY
kills time	makes time
makes promises	makes commitments
controls	empowers
resents others	learns from others
I'll try that	I'll do that
sees problems	sees opportunities
wishes	makes dreams come true
expects to fail	expects to succeed
is part of the problem	is part of the solution

As Pauline Mowat, aged 83 and a Mental Fitness for Life workshop participant, wrote:

> My goal was to use the language of possibility when referring to old age. And I have realized that I can be in charge of my language and my attitude rather than drifting with the environment and responding to circumstances. I can feel an inner strength that is real, expected, and permanent. It is not a self-analysis game, involving cause and effect. It just is. In fact, it always was but I hadn't noticed. It is like a pillar of strength that is me. There is no pride in this discovery, no self-consciousness, just fact. A very humbling fact. It does not involve trying to be anything, trying to prove anything or competing with anything. It is a great big freedom to be myself and be happy about it. If one can be pronounced physically fit, can I be pronounced mentally fit? What has helped me is coming to the classes, all the people, the freedom of expression and that feeling that I could do anything here.

Critical thinking skills were used effectively in the Mental Fitness Pilot Program as a technique to challenge the assumptions that people have about aging that limit their options for a healthy old age, and changing negative beliefs to positive beliefs about the limitless possibilities for growth and development in later life. The challenge is to create a new perspective of old age by changing our belief systems based on new research in aging that is more hopeful and optimistic.

People in the program were empowered to change. They were given the support and the encouragement they needed to make dramatic changes in the way they felt and thought about themselves and their skills and abilities. They increased awareness about how habitual ways of thinking and being controlled their thinking and what they were able to achieve. The first group of people (between the ages of 63 and 83) completed the Mental Fitness Pilot Program in December 1996. Evaluation research provides evidence of improved mental fitness knowledge and skills, and changed attitudes, beliefs, and behaviors. Many claimed a new awareness of how their thoughts control their actions, and a shift from negative to positive thinking about themselves and others. They were empowered: they were given the inspiration, the motivation, the will, and the support they needed to achieve more than they had ever dreamed possible.

Barbara Guttmann-Gee is a woman 88 years of age; she grew up in Britain and was accepted at Oxford at the age of 16. However, the Depression and World War II intervened in her studies. She married and emigrated to Canada, where she worked in secretarial jobs most of her life. When she retired, she enrolled in the Open Learning Institute and received a B.A. in her 70s, then an M.A. in Women's Studies from Simon Fraser University at 81. Physically, she fits the stereotype of the "sweet little old lady"—but like all stereotypes, it fails to convey the richness of her experience, her sharp mind, and her ability to speak her mind eloquently when the opportunity arises. She enrolled in the mental fitness class because she felt she was getting mentally and physically lazy and needed something to get her back on track: she wanted to gain confidence and new knowledge to fuel her keen interest in destroying the myth that "mental faculties decline with age."

Before she undertook university studies, she believed that her mental faculties would diminish with age, but research for a master's degree together with personal experience changed this belief. Her mental ability continues to improve because she has a desire to keep her mind active.

Barbara's personal mental fitness goal was to build more confidence and knowledge to support her mission in life, which is to foster education for older people. As part of her goal, she spoke to a group of students at the university who are studying how to teach older people. She spoke about her experiences as a senior student, and was very critical of the quality of instruction at the university. She gave students tips to improve instruction for older adults and impressed them with her spirit of adventure.

When asked to give the mental fitness class an update on her goals and achievements, she reported that she had been interviewed on television:

Last week I was a guest on a TV show entitled Generations. *I was asked to speak about the importance of learning, and why I was driven to go back to school and get a B.A. and then an M.A. And I spoke of the mental fitness program and how I was learning about new research that suggests the brain doesn't deteriorate when you get older. When you get older, there can be a lot of "clutter in the attic," but you just have to get rid of it. If you let your muscles go, they deteriorate, and the same is true for the brain. In fact, to be fair, something vital may go, but the brain can still remain active. In other words, mental fitness doesn't solve all the problems of aging. But if you are doing a course, you have a goal, something that drives you on, and you forget your aches and pains. This class has helped me enormously. It has given me the push, it got the adrenaline going again, and I was able to make more progress.*

Barbara was able to achieve her lifelong goals, to live her lifelong dreams, and to leave a legacy for others through the example of her life. The mental fitness program helped her to build confidence and stay focused. She received an honorary doctorate for her contribution.

🖉 ASSIGNMENT: OPTIONAL BUT CRITICAL

1. Tune in to people's language, particularly negative or limiting words. This will heighten your awareness.
2. Listen to your own words. Buy an eraser and carry it with you. Every time you hear yourself use a negative or limiting word, take the eraser out and erase those words out of your mind. Then replace the negative words with positive ones.
3. Now let's return to the newspaper article on page 82 and, using your new thinking tools, identify any negative, limiting language. What are the limiting beliefs that are reflected in the language?

3

STEP

CREATIVITY:
OUT *of* THE BOX *and* OVER *the* MOON

Creativity is as essential to your survival as breathing.

—TONY BUZAN

We deliberated about whether the third component of mental fitness should be "creative thinking" or "creativity." Creative thinking seemed the more logical next step in a mental fitness program. But logic is not what creativity is all about. Ultimately, Gene Cohen's brilliant book *The Creative Age* convinced us that Step 3 should be called simply Creativity.

What would you say if we asked you, "Are you creative?" or "How creative do you think you are?" Most people answer, "I'm not creative." It is our beliefs about creativity that keep us from developing our full creative potential. And believe it or not, you are about to discover how creative you really are.

There is a great deal of controversy about creativity. What does it mean? Are you born with it? Is your IQ higher if you have more of it? Can creativity be learned? Nurtured? Enhanced? How important is it? Do so-called creative people have the edge? Why should you want to be creative? What are the benefits? How will it help in your daily life? How is it related to keeping your mind sharp? To health? To aging? When was the last time you used your creative powers? How old were you? When were you last given an opportunity to be creative and to think creatively? What did you create? These are the questions many people ask, and this chapter is filled with answers—and more. So let's dig in and explore the mystery of creativity. But first, some exercises to warm up your creative thinking skills and stretch your mind in new directions.

🤸 WARM-UP EXERCISES

EXERCISE 1: **THE MYSTERY PARAGRAPH**

How quickly can you find out what is so unusual about this paragraph? It looks so ordinary that you would think that nothing was wrong with it at all and, in fact, nothing is. But it is unusual. Why? If you study it and think about it you may find out but I am not going to assist you in any way. You must do it without coaching. No doubt, if you work at it for long, it will dawn on you. Who knows? Go to work and try your skill. Par is about half an hour. (See "Clues and Answers," page 240.)

EXERCISE 2: **THE RIVER PROBLEM**

A man wishes to cross a wide, deep river, as shown in the diagram. There is no bridge, no boat, and he cannot swim. How does he get across?

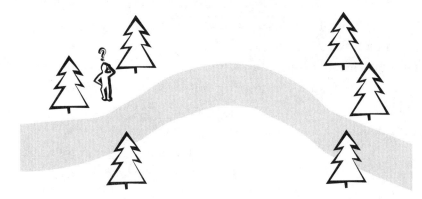

EXERCISE 3: **BLINDED AT TEATIME**

A man was drinking a cup of tea when he was suddenly blinded. How?

(For the answers to these exercises, see "Clues and Answers," page 240–41.)

Creativity has so many different meanings, and we use so many different words to describe it. Some meanings will jump out at you; some won't. Read carefully through this chapter from beginning to end. When theory and experience are carefully interwoven, the words have the power to transform your thinking and your life.

Here's some creative fun to get us going—one person's view of what would happen if we started to live our life backwards.

A wealthy woman asked a famous millinery designer to design a hat for her. He placed a canvas form on her head, and in eight minutes with a single piece of ribbon, he created a beautiful hat right before her eyes. The matron was delighted.

"How much will that be?" she asked.

"Fifty dollars," he replied.

"Why, that's outrageous," she said, "It's only a piece of ribbon!"

The milliner quickly unraveled the ribbon and, handing it to her, said, "Madame, the ribbon is free."

—ABIGAIL VAN BUREN

Reverse Living

Life is tough. It takes up a lot of your time, all your weekends, and what do you get at the end of it? Death, a great reward.

I think that the life cycle is all backwards. You should die first, get it out of the way, then you live 20 years in an old age home. You get kicked out when you're too young, you get a gold watch, you go to work. You work 40 years until you're young enough to enjoy your retirement.

You go to college, you do drugs, you do alcohol, you party, until you're ready for high school, you go to grade school, you become a little kid, you play, you have no responsibilities, you become a little baby, you go back into the womb, you spend your last nine months floating, and you finish off as a gleam in somebody's eye.

—ROGER VON OECH

Generally speaking, creativity is a mystery to people and its many and various definitions help to keep it that way. Even the way you think about creativity is an indication of your creativity. You may be thinking, "Why should I bother being creative or thinking creatively?" In the past, we were taught that creativity was a rare gift; people are born with it— artists, musicians, painters, composers, writers. Maybe you said to yourself, "That's not me." We now know creativity goes well beyond the arts, and young and old alike have more than a spark of creativity in them. Most people just need a jump-start; that's what we plan to give you in this chapter.

> The **mind**, once **stretched** by a **new idea**, never regains its **original dimension**.
>
> —OLIVER WENDELL HOLMES

Imagine someone getting out the red and black heavy-duty battery cables, squeezing open the clasp and clamping them to the sides of your head, turning the key in the ignition and—

wham—a jolt of creative current jump-starts your mind. All sorts of things will begin to happen. One of the first things that will happen is that you begin to rid yourself of lessons you learned as a child.

Do any of the following sound familiar?

"You can't color over the line."
"*That's* a tea pot?"
"The sky isn't green!"
"You can be in the choir, but just mouth the words."
"We've never done it that way before."
"Can you make your picture look more like Johnny's?"
"How can I tell that's a cow?"

If those lessons didn't drive the creativity right out of you, how about these instructions:

"Don't be foolish, be realistic."
"You must follow the rules."
"Don't draw attention to yourself."
"Quit daydreaming."
"Don't be so silly."

Did you feel your creativity shutting down? Do you remember feeling ashamed? Nowadays we call it being boxed in—and what keeps us in the box is the negative attitudes that undermine our creativity.

I stood up in my first grade class and said, "Do these chairs have to be in rows? Can we put them in a circle, or sit on the floor?" The answer was no, and I began to hide my creative thinking. I also began to invent illnesses so that I could stay home from school and read, write and create. One year, I missed 92 days. I believe that this saved my creative life. —SARK

One reason we resist so vigorously the idea of growing older is that we have been led to believe that old age is the end of both mental and creative accomplishments. A theoretical perspective, based on a review of the literature, will help you to understand where those negative attitudes came from, why they are no longer valid, and, finally, how to exercise your creativity and reap all the benefits. You are already an authority on your own life experience, and once you have an understanding of what the experts have said about creativity in general, you can become an expert on your own creativity.

Believe it or not, people have been doing research on creativity for at least 500 years. Until the mid-20th century, studies suggested that creativity is the prerogative of youth, while age means a decline in creative powers. One study covered a 150-year period (from 1835 to 1969) and examined the careers of artists and scientists in order to chart productivity. The findings showed that there were a few older artists who were still producing artwork, but generally speaking, creativity declines with age.

The belief that people become less creative as they age was hotly debated at the turn of the 20th century. In 1905, the great orator Sir William Osler claimed that the effective, vitalizing work of the world is accomplished between the ages of 25 and 40. Those 15 golden years were identified as the productive period when most artists and scientists create their most important work.

Public debate raged around this issue, with one side agreeing with Osler that creative ability is the province of the young and the other claiming that creativity is a human trait present throughout the life course and is undiminished or even increased by chronological age.

This debate continued through the 20th century. Studies generally indicated that the creative energies of an artist were destined to dry up, and that the greatest tragedy for the aging poet, painter, novelist, or playwright is the growing inability to express them- selves creatively. One study describes the personal experience of a woman who struggles to live, love, and write to the utmost while she is young because she feels that when her energy is gone, she will regret all she hasn't created. How sad to hold such limiting beliefs in our creative energy!

If the general belief in society is that chronological age brings loss of creativity and inevitable decline, many people will be denied the opportunity to use their abilities, without regard to how well they function or to the amount of useful knowledge they possess— for no other reason than their chronological age.

Now, in the early years of the 21st century, we have powerful new evidence that the creative spirit is a source of unlimited energy and vitality. The proponents of these two opposing views about cre- ativity—is it or isn't it reduced with age—still vie for our attention today. Until the mistaken assumptions are openly refuted, the belief in inevitable decline with age will continue to have a powerful neg- ative impact on millions of people.

CAN OLDER PEOPLE BE CREATIVE?

Yes. Henry Wadsworth Longfellow thought so. His poem "Morituri Salutamus" honors creative older people of the past.

> *Cato learned Greek at eighty; Sophocles*
> *Wrote his grand "Oedipus," and Simonides*
> *Bore off the prize of verse from his compeers,*
> *When each had numbered more than fourscore years;*
> *And Theophrastus, at four score and ten,*
> *Had begun his "Characters of Men."*

Chaucer, at Woodstock, with the nightingales,
At sixty wrote the "Canterbury Tales."
Goethe, at Weimar, toiling to the last,
Completed "Faust" when eighty years were past. . . .

What is unique and positive at the beginning of the 21st century is that we now have the research to lay the negative assumptions to rest *once and for all.* The work of Gene Cohen provides strong evidence that everyone can be creative and creative accomplishments do not decline with age.

> No **great** thing is **created** suddenly, any more than a bunch of grapes or a fig. If you tell me that you **desire** a fig, I answer you that there **must be time.** Let it first blossom, then **bear fruit,** then ripen.
> —EPICTETUS

Cohen argues that, as we age, creativity is largely undermined by negative attitudes. Fatigue, lack of motivation, and senility—explanations that are offered for the decline in artistic productivity over time—are all based on false assumptions about general decline with age. Artists mature with age and often produce their most important work in later life. World-famous masterpieces are not identified as "by Rembrandt, age 75." Think about it: age is irrelevant.

ARE YOU CREATIVE?

The second important question is this: Can anyone be creative? Again, Cohen argues that creativity is not just for the gifted few, and he also provides a definition of creativity that serves as a blueprint for how to develop your own creativity. He defines creativity as "the innate capacity for growth, the energy that allows us to think a different thought or express ourselves in a novel way."

WHAT *Is* CREATIVITY *and* HOW DO WE DEVELOP IT?

Gene Cohen developed what he calls the creative equation:

$C = me^2$

C = creativity

m = mass of knowledge

e = experience

2 = two types of experience

    1. *inner* emotional experience

    2. *external* life experience

Creativity equals our mass of knowledge multiplied by our two types of experience (inner and external). This means that our creative potential increases with age. If, for example, we assume that as we age our mass of knowledge increases, then if everything else in the equation remains the same, the creative score increases by virtue of longevity alone. If we assume that one's emotional experience deepens with age, then by virtue of enriched emotional experience alone, one's creativity would increase. To put it another way, as our knowledge increases and our emotional experience deepens and our life experience increases, we become more creative. That means that all of us, no matter what age, can take hold of this promise and exercise creativity as long as we live.

THE CREATIVE AGE

We are living in a creative age in which innovation and creativity are prized in every area of life, from business to personal relationships. And, according to Cohen, the phase of life beyond the age of 50 years is the most creative phase of one's life. He has categorized four stages of creativity:

1. The re-evaluation phase, which begins in our 50s when creative expression is intensified by a sense of crisis or quest
2. The liberation phase, beginning in our 60s or 70s, when creative endeavors are charged with new energy brought about by retirement or change in workload
3. The summing-up phase, from the 70s on, which focuses on looking back, summing up, and giving back
4. The encore phase, from the 80s onward, which focuses on affirming life and making a contribution

No matter what age or phase you are in, you can develop your full creative potential. But first, it's time for a quick review:

WHAT WE KNOW *About* CREATIVITY

- Creativity is not the privilege of youth. There are many examples of great achievements in every field by people who are very old.
- People may, in fact, make their greatest creative contribution in later life.
- If you believe that your creativity will diminish as you get older, it probably will.
- No more theoretical arguments: the evidence is in, and it's time to get creative.

HOW *to* GET CREATIVE

One of the most helpful activities to jump-start creative thinking and drive home the concept is the well-known "connect the dots" exercise. It comes from the work of Mike Vance and Diane Deacon in their book *Think Out of the Box.*

EXERCISE 4: **CONNECT THE DOTS**

Take a few minutes to connect the dots.
  1. Connect all nine dots using no more than four straight lines.
  2. The dots cannot be repositioned.
  3. The connecting line must be drawn in one continuous stroke.
  4. Leave the pencil on the paper until all lines have been drawn.

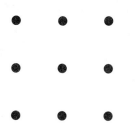

(See the solution in "Clues and Answers," page 242.)
The concept here is to allow our thinking to branch out—not to be contained or limited by imaginary boundaries. Mental barriers limit our ability and prevent us from "getting out of the box." Thinking outside of the box is what creative thinking is all about.

I'm walking to work up Sixth Avenue and it's a lovely spring day and I see one of those mime performers. So the mime is doing that famous routine where he's pretending to be trapped in a box. So I stand there and watch the mime pretend to be trapped in a box. And he finishes up, and thank God, he wasn't really trapped in a box. And I see on the sidewalk there he's got a little hat for money—change, tips, donations, contributions. So I walk over and I pretend to put a dollar bill in his hat.

—DAVID LETTERMAN

Webster's Dictionary defines creativity as (1) the quality of being creative, and (2) the ability to create. So, are you creative? How can you tell? Do tests really tell us how creative we are? Or do they simply tell us how creative we aren't? Here is the best test we have found.

Are you creative? (check the appropriate box)

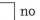 yes   no

In Roger von Oech's excellent book *A Whack on the Side of the Head,* he tells the story of a major company that was concerned about the lack of creative productivity among some of the personnel. The management brought in a team of psychologists to find out why some people were more creative than others. By doing this they hoped they could stimulate the "less creative people." The psychologists studied the group for three months, asking questions that ranged from their educational backgrounds to their favorite color. What they discovered was the following: the creative people thought they were creative and the less creative people didn't think they were.

People who don't think they are creative often stifle themselves because they have not fully explored what creativity can mean to them. They often make excuses for their seeming lack of creativity by claiming that creativity belongs only to the Mozarts and Einsteins of the world. But they are wrong—consider the story of the two frogs:

Humor is liberating. Use it liberally. It loosens the muscles and frees the mind to make new connections.

—GENE COHEN

The Two Frogs

Once upon a time, two frogs fell into a bucket of cream. The first frog, seeing that there was no way to get any footing in the white liquid, accepted his fate and drowned. The second frog didn't like that approach. He started thrashing around in the cream and doing whatever he could to stay afloat. After a while, all of his churning turned the cream into butter, and he was able to hop out.

—ROGER VON OECH

Moral of the story: even a frog can be creative.

Creativity and the Performing Arts

This is how the great modern dancer Martha Graham thinks about creativity:

There is a vitality, a life force, a quickening that is translated through you into action and because there is only one of you in all time, this expression is unique. And if you block it, it will never exist through any other medium and be lost. The world will not have it. It is not your business to determine how good it is, nor how valuable it is, nor how it compares with other expressions. It is your business to keep it yours clearly and directly, and to keep the channel open. You do not even have to believe in yourself or your work. You have to keep open and aware directly to the urges that motivate you. There is no satisfaction whatever at any time. There is only queer dissatisfaction; a blessed unrest that keeps us marching and makes us more alive than others.

Martha Graham refers to the creative spirit as a restless anxiety that must be expressed. Surely, you may say, that feeling is characteristic of the creative geniuses (poets, musicians, dancers, actors) among us who earn their living by their craft. Wrong. We all have creativity within us—all we have to do is find a way to use it and benefit from the energy that may manifest as anxiety just waiting to be released. It makes sense to harness our anxieties into creative endeavor because it gives us energy and vitality. After all, it is how people of all ages, of all intellects, of all colors, cultures, and creeds have developed incredible means of survival.

> Creativity is there all the time. We're the ones who leave it. We wait for the inspiration to start, yet it's really the other way round—first the action, then the inspiration.
>
> —SARK

During the Depression of the 1930s people "made do" with very little; they created meals for large families from nothing. For dessert? Soda crackers in water with a dab of brown sugar on top. It takes more creativity to "dream up" something from nothing than to create a gourmet meal today. Recently we were at a friend's house and she showed us a set of end tables, the legs of which were made by her great-grandmother out of sewing spools piled and glued on top of each other. Now, that's creativity.

The distinguished American gerontologist and noted scholar Robert Kastenbaum refers to creativity as "serious play and infinite limits." His definition is this:

Creativity is an attitude and a process that sometimes—but not invariably—results in a palpable outcome or product. Creativity as an attitude asserts, "This is a fresh moment: I can help bring something new into the world." Creativity as a process demands, "Be open to all influences, inner and outer. Experience clearly, keenly, intensely. Now work like a demon! Now step back and inspect like a critic. Now work again!" The outcome could be a recognizable "thing" such as a piece of furniture, an invention, a blueprint, a poem, a song. Or the outcome could be less tangible though not less real: a group's altered image of itself, a long-term relationship taken a new and exciting turn, an individual's lifestyle transformed into both a deeper and a more spontaneous communion with inner and outer reality. Creativity is both the instantaneous spark of inspiration and the long, strenuous effort to bring that idea to fulfillment.

Anxiety is the handmaiden of **creativity.**

—CHUCK JONES

Creativity takes many different forms. If we stretch our minds beyond everyday habits of thinking, we can come up with numerous examples of the creative spirit. Like we've said, part of the challenge is overcoming the idea that creativity is restricted to creating a piece of art—a painting or a sculpture—or composing a piece of music. We have believed that genius like Mozart's, is well beyond our reach. Creative writing is for the specially gifted and, besides, creative people are born with it, we think.

Adversity reveals genius, prosperity conceals it.

—HORACE

In today's society, thanks to creative thinking, creativity is taking on new meaning. We are now in the Creative Age. Creative cooks, creative thinkers, creative employees are sought by creative employers. Creativity tests have been created to hire creative, innovative thinkers. Humor is a creative endeavor. Even though for most people writing letters is a lost art, when we unleash our mind, we can write letters like never before—as Aunt Ethel did:

Dear Carl,

I'm writing this slow because I know you can't read fast. We don't live where we did when you left. Your Dad read in the paper that most accidents happen within twenty miles of home, so we moved. I can't send you the address as the family that lived here before took the numbers with them for their next house, so they wouldn't have to change their address.

This place has a washing machine but the first day I put four shirts in it and pulled the chain. Guess what—I haven't seen them since.

It rained here only twice last week, three days the first time and four the second.

About the coat you want me to send you. Aunt Mabel said it would be a little too heavy to send in the mail with them heavy buttons, so we cut them off and hid them in the pocket.

We got a bill from the Funeral Home and they said that if we didn't make the payments on old Aunt Bessie's funeral—up she comes.

We hear you had a new baby recently—please let me know right away whether it's a girl or boy so I'll know if I'm an aunt or uncle.

Your Uncle John fell into the Whiskey Vat. Some men

tried to pull him out but he fought them off and drowned. We cremated him and he burned for three days.

Three of your friends went off the bridge in their pickup. One was driving and the other two drowned because they couldn't get the tail gate open.

Aunt Isabel is knitting you some socks. She would have sent them by now but I told her you had grown another foot since she last saw you so she is busy knitting another one.

Not much news this time as nothing much has happened here.

Love, Aunt Ethel

In many ways, creativity is underrated—it's not just painting or writing. Creativity includes talent, skills, challenges, imagination, personality, values, motivations. We can learn about creativity and we can experience creativity—but we don't necessarily approach it in a logical way. You discover creativity by experiencing it yourself. You will take from this chapter and the book what you will: some things will work for you; some will not.

> Don't think! Thinking is the enemy of creativity. It's self-conscious and anything self-conscious is lousy. You can't try to do things. You simply must do things.
>
> —RAY BRADBURY

Perhaps the best we can do is to dip into the well with our own unique bucket, draw something up that is normally beyond our reach, and make something happen. Not everyone agrees with all these ideas. Nonetheless, creativity started the world and it's here to stay. Everyone is creative whether they think they are or not, and each one will choose to explore creativity in his or her own way.

Different Forms of Creativity

It's time to shed some light on the distinctions between creativity, creative thinking, and creative self-expression. People mean different ent things when they speak and write about creativity. Here are some important distinctions:

We exercise our creativity when we engage in any one of its myriad forms of expression. Basically, creativity means bringing something new into existence. In fact, it is possible to create even without writing a word or painting a picture—by simply (and perhaps most profoundly) molding one's inner life.

Creative thinking involves breaking away from logical ways of thinking and using imagination, intuition, and dreams, which give us new ideas and ways to look at things without judging, censoring, or stifling. It may involve breaking rules and established patterns that inhibit us at every turn. We are then better able to solve everyday problems.

> In the creative state a man is taken out of himself. He lets down as it were a bucket into his subconscious, and draws up something which is normally beyond his reach. He mixes his thinking with his normal experiences and out of the mixture he makes a work of art.
>
> —E.M. FORSTER

Seasoned actor Joy Coghill suggests that long life provides the opportunity to make a unique and important contribution to society. She founded Western Gold Theatre, a company made up of senior performing artists, because she felt that these artists were not only wiser and richer in experience than they were at 40 or 50, but they had something to say that was fresh, unique, challenging, and entertaining. And when that contribution is an expression of one's unique talents and skills, the creative self-expression itself is life-enhancing.

It's **never too late** to be what you **might** have been.

—GEORGE ELIOT

While Coghill's experience is with professional performing artists, creative self-expression can be found anywhere. You can express creativity through knitting. Or through golf, if you practice it as a creative art or as a meditation. It all depends on whether you do it with your whole person—body, mind, and spirit. And the benefits of creative expression, the renewal of energy and vitality, work for everyone.

The creative spirit never dies nor diminishes with age, unless we block it or kill it. Creativity is blocked when we ignore it, devalue it, or anesthetize it by mindless activity (for example, watching TV). The image in Chekhov's play *The Seagull* springs to mind. The stuffed seagull sits on the mantel, expression glazed, while people play cards, people who suffer from laziness, apathy, and the limiting beliefs drilled into them since childhood about what they can and cannot do.

Ultimately, we are limited only by the limitations we place on ourselves. In fact, one can accomplish far more in that last third of life simply because there's no time to become "perfect," so you just go for it! It doesn't matter if it suits others, for it is in the doing that your soul becomes enriched and your spirit soars. When that spirit is expressed through live performance, the benefits go far beyond the artists. What is even more extraordinary is that the experience of attending a live performance has a positive impact on the health and well-being of the audience.

If attending live theater engages the audience in a way that gives people a vitality and energy and sense of well-being that is missing in mediated performance (TV and film), consider the implications. Doctors could prescribe a night at the opera, rather than expensive medications with debilitating side effects. In addition, the positive emotional state that results from live performance (increased self-esteem, personal mastery, feelings of optimism) can motivate people to adopt a more healthy lifestyle. Furthermore, new evidence suggests that positive emotional states can strengthen the immune, neural, and endocrine systems as well.

Time for another review. What is creativity?

Creativity is . . .
- designing a uniquely beautiful item of clothing.
- a new way of looking at life that is humorous.
- arranging the chairs in a room differently.
- solving problems in a new way.
- pantomime, creative thinking, and humor.
- dancing.
- creating a gourmet meal.
- a unique response to adversity.
- composing a piece of music.

As Tony Buzan has stated, "Creativity is as essential to survival as breathing." It allows you to be flexible and inventive in your approach to all kinds of problems. Creativity helps you to adapt to changes spontaneously; it releases stress and improves enjoyment in life. There are numerous other benefits to developing creative ways to live life. Once you are aware of the possibilities stored within you, you will be free to explore experiences you may have only dreamed of. Like anything new, creativity can be viewed as a skill instead of an innate gift. Creativity can be learned and nurtured and enhanced.

Why should you want to be creative?

Why Be Creative?

- Creative people solve problems.
- Creative people don't fear the future; they look forward to the challenges that change brings.
- Creativity is good for your health.
- Creative people have a competitive advantage.
- There is a great need for "out of the box" thinking in the world today.

> The end of every maker
> is himself.
> —ST. THOMAS AQUINAS

The walls of ageism are being torn down, brick by brick, with each example of an older person accomplishing, contributing, enjoying, changing, growing, creating new facets of life. We can look for inspiration to the widely recognized creativity of people like Georgia O'Keeffe or George Burns. We can look closer to home, in our communities, where new contributions and friendships result from intergenerational creativity. Finally, we can look inward, and . . . find in ourselves the capacity for creative growth and expression that can uplift our lives and inspire others. . . . Our willingness to embrace the challenge and the opportunity will define the legacy that each of us builds, and the gift that each of us gives, in every season of our lives.

—GENE COHEN

The argument won't be closed until we no longer marvel at the creative accomplishments of people who are very old. Then we will have succeeded in making the point—and there will no longer be the need to present our evidence.

Finally, before we give you some suggestions on how you can exercise your creative powers, here is a testimonial from one of our mental fitness program participants:

"Getting Out of the Box" by Jo Ebert, age 85

The expression "getting out of the box" is used everywhere these days, even in the business world, and it is an outcome of our creative thinking. Creativity is an attribute of every human being, not just the gifted. It is an expression of the human spirit, and when our creative mind encourages us to explore new avenues in life, we are helping ourselves to get rid of the negative myths that have boxed us in over the years; myths such as the belief that mental and physical capacities inevitably decline as we age. This is patently not true, and thinking this way prevents us from enjoying life as much as we should. So, I am going to tell you a couple of stories about how I got out of the box.

My first really exciting experience in getting out of the box occurred a few years ago when I attended a play by Morris Panych called *The History of Things to Come*. As you can tell by the title, it was a very obscure play, and I didn't understand any of it. But at one point in the play, the leading character asked for volunteers from the audience. Because I was only four rows from the stage, I knew I would have a very good chance of being picked. And sure enough I was. I went up onto the stage and was led to the wings where I was given a regal costume with a crown and I was led out onto the stage. The actors began asking me questions. Finally, one asked: "How did you get to be King?" And I told them: "I never was until I was kidnapped by you people." I think he thought I might steal the show, because he promptly ushered me into the wings.

In creating, the only hard thing is to begin; a grass-blade's no easier to make than an oak.

—JAMES RUSSELL LOWELL

I was so pleased with myself. It was a wonderful experience. I would never have had the courage to do it if I hadn't been attending mental fitness classes. These classes give us many opportunities to speak out before the group and we get lots of support and encouragement. This boosts our self-esteem so we are fairly comfortable embarking on new ventures.

So you see, getting out of the box is very rewarding and if I can do these things at 84, it's never too late for you. And you don't have to wait as long as I did to have this kind of fun.

Jo Ebert was born in New Zealand in 1917 and came to Canada when she was five years old. She graduated from St. Paul's Hospital nursing program and has been an enthusiastic member of our mental fitness class for many years. Her cheerfulness and humor have helped to make each class more enjoyable. She says we are going to miss her when she leaves us at 102.

When you are completely **absorbed** or caught up in something, you **become oblivious** of things around you, or of the **passage of time**. It is this absorption in what you are doing that frees your **unconscious** and **releases** **your creative imagination.**

—ROLLO MAY

IT'S YOUR TURN *to* GET CREATIVE

This section is not a step-by-step guide to creativity guaranteed or your money back. That's impossible. On the other hand, creativity should not be left to take care of itself. We can't promise the Sistine Chapel, but we can promise a way to think differently about the creativity that lies within each of us—that defines us and creates a happier, more fulfilled way of life. We are hoping you will make exploring your creativity one of your most important goals. What follows are numerous suggestions and ideas that you can pick from to start tapping into your hidden creative self or to nurture and enhance the creativity that you are already aware of and expressing.

🐝 EXERCISING YOUR CREATIVE POWERS

1. Start your own personal creativity development program.
2. Try a new style of dress.
3. Make time to play with children and with the child within you.
4. Read creativity books. (We highly recommend *The Creative Age* by Gene Cohen and Tony Buzan's *Book of Genius*.)
5. Make friends with people of all ages and backgrounds.
6. Work on solving problems instead of worrying about them.
7. Develop your sense of humor; learn to tell a joke.
8. Start or continue to write poetry.
9. Develop your artistic skills—join a drama group, take a drawing class.
10. Change your vocabulary; eliminate negative words and replace them with positive ones.
11. Read books on various subjects.
12. Learn about something new that you know absolutely nothing about.
13. Play unfamiliar music. Perhaps the different vibrations stimulate the brain in new ways. Some people play Mozart for babies because it makes them more creative. Try playing Mozart and see if it makes you feel more intelligent and more creative.
14. Jot down wild ideas when they pop into your mind.
15. Don't be afraid to fall in love with something or someone and pursue it with passion.

16. Know and take pride in, practice, develop, use, and enjoy your greatest strengths. (Everyone has a special gift or talent that is just waiting to be unleashed.)
17. Find a great teacher or mentor who will help you.
18. Don't waste a lot of expensive, unproductive energy trying to be "well-rounded"; focus on what you do well and what you are passionate about.
19. Make a treasure hunt for your adult friends.
20. Surround yourself with happy memories, photos that make you tingle. Change them around every month.
21. Make that long hallway in your house an art gallery.
22. Make up your own puzzles and clues and try them at your next party.
23. Sit alone, think only pleasant thoughts, feel the peace, and let your mind start to create.

People often say that this or that person has not yet found himself. But the self is not something that one finds. It is something that one creates.

—THOMAS SZASZ

These are just a few ideas to push you closer to your creative edge. There are other books full of ideas—but your own brain has more than enough to last a lifetime. We'd like to leave you with the knowledge that you, too, can be a creative genius. Tony Buzan talks about psychologists who have studied Mozart's life and identified him as "psychotically positive" because his letters to his wife were so extremely optimistic.

In the early 1990s psychologists studying Mozart's letters revealed a finding that they considered most odd: they had "discovered" that Mozart was, to use their jargon, "psychotically positive." They misnamed him this because they had found a letter in which he had written to his wife that a new opening performance of one of his operas had gone exceptionally well. Mozart had happily described all the positive aspects of the performance, mentioning only at the end that it had not met with critical acclaim, and that the audience had numbered only 10 people!

Mozart, like most other leading geniuses, intuitively realized that it was far more productive for creative processes and musical composition to focus on excellence rather than to dwell on the negative. He was, contrary to the psychologists' assumptions, appropriately positive. In his honor, Tony Buzan calls creativity + optimism the Amadeity Principle.

We hope that we have convinced you that you can be creative—even more so than you are now—and that all you have to do is to exercise your creative powers. In the next chapter, we'll take you beyond the Amadeity Principle, demonstrating how to become and remain optimistic in your journey through life and time. Make yourself a promise that you are going to live more fully, more creatively, and more passionately every day of your life.

ASSIGNMENT

Just for fun write a four-line poem—a funny one—and share it with someone. It could be a rhyme like:

> *I saw the sunset glow*
> *Peeking through a distant mountain row*
> *Still, still, the wind stood still*
> *Ruined by a cackling crow.*

That took 30 seconds. Even if you hate poetry, or if you just don't feel like doing it—do it anyway—it will release some creative juices.

STEP 4

POSITIVE MENTAL ATTITUDE

The greatest revolution of my life is the discovery that individuals can change the outer aspects of their lives by changing the inner attitudes of their minds.

—WILLIAM JAMES

T his chapter is about mental attitude: what it is, why it's important, and how to develop a positive mental attitude. Webster's Dictionary defines attitude as a way of acting, feeling, or thinking; one's disposition or outlook. It is a frame of mind affecting one's thoughts and behavior. The word optimism is derived from the Latin *optimum*, meaning best, and is defined as an inclination to expect the best possible outcome. Our mental fitness definition would simply be that developing a positive mental attitude means putting a favorable spin on everything and expecting the best. The great Roman poet Horace put it this way, "What shall be tomorrow, think not of asking. Each day that Fortune gives you, be it what it may, set down for gain."

What are the advantages and benefits of having a positive mental attitude (PMA)? What does the research tell us? What can you do to increase your level of optimism, and what can you do to maintain it? What role does hope play? In the pages that follow, we intend to convince you that the most important thing any of us can do for our mind and health is to develop an attitude of optimism.

But first, here is your mental fitness warm-up. Each of the 12 items in the first exercise is a separate puzzle. How many can you figure out on your own? If you get stuck, try them out on a friend. See "Clues and Answers," page 242, for the solutions.

MENTAL FITNESS WARM-UP

EXERCISE 1

PAID I'M WORKED	*LIBRARY* *LIBRARY*	DON'T / DO IT	JUST *144* ICE
1	2	3	4
pay pay	A MTOWNN	KJUSTK	CAST CAST CAST CAST
5	6	7	8
TOR / TOE	gettingitall	G W / N E / I D D	ERIF
9	10	11	12

Bring to this puzzle the attitude that you expect to solve it and see what happens. Even if you don't solve it, you'll likely have fun trying.

EXERCISE 2: The Miller's Daughter

Many years ago, there was a poor miller who could not afford to pay the rent on his mill. His grasping old landlord threatened to evict him, his wife, and his daughter. However, the landlord did offer an option. If the miller's beautiful young daughter would marry the old man, he would forget their debts and let the miller and his wife live in the mill rent-free.

The family met to discuss this offer. The daughter was horrified at the prospect of marriage to the old man, but she realized that it might be the only hope for her parents. She suggested a compromise. They would draw lots. If the landlord won, she would meet his request and if she won, he would wipe out all debts without her having to marry him. The landlord agreed.

The two stood on a stony path that had many black and white pebbles. The landlord suggested that they put one black pebble and one white pebble in the bag. If the black one was chosen, she must marry him; if it was white, she would be free. She agreed to this suggestion. He bent down and picked up two pebbles to put in the bag, but she noticed he had cheated and put in two black pebbles.

She could expose him by showing that there were now two black pebbles in the bag, but he would lose face in front of all the people and might evict them in his anger. How could she seem to go along with the plan and win, knowing that there were two black pebbles in the bag?

OPTIMISM AS *the* FREEDOM *to* CHOOSE

No discussion of positive attitude would be complete without mentioning one of the most remarkable human beings of the last century. In his book *Man's Search for Meaning*, Dr. Viktor Frankl writes about his three years in the Nazi concentration camps of Auschwitz and Dachau. He describes the trauma and suffering that he and others endured. He describes witnessing his friends and relatives being buried alive or herded into gas chambers. Somehow, he survived the living nightmare of starvation and torture. What is so remarkable about Viktor Frankl is what he learned. This is the message he left for us:

> *We who lived in concentration camps can remember the men who walked through the huts comforting others, giving away their last piece of bread. They may have been few in number, but they offer sufficient proof that our mind determines our attitude. That everything can be taken from a man but one thing: the last of the human freedoms—to choose one's attitude in any given set of circumstances, to choose one's own way. And there were always choices to make. Every day, every hour, offered the opportunity to make a decision, a decision which determined whether you would or would not submit to those powers which threatened to rob you of your very self, your inner freedom. . . .*

The survivors of Auschwitz and Dachau were those who maintained the freedom to choose, an attitude that helped them get through every hour, every minute. If Frankl had choices, so do we. We can take the pessimistic view or we can take the optimistic view—the position of hopefulness that believes this too will pass, and the best is yet to come.

Many people think of themselves as being optimistic without really understanding what it means. That was certainly true for us until we researched the topic more thoroughly. Many people use clichés such as "Never give up" or "Never say die" or "When the going gets tough, the tough get going." While these are great mottoes to live by, they don't necessarily speak to the essence of optimism. We're going to take you on a journey into the heart of the matter.

Many excellent books have been written about positive mental attitude, and this chapter incorporates some that have influenced our work. The topic is so important that it probably should be our starting point, because everything in life, including getting mentally fit, is based on our attitude. We place it here for a reason—we know now that you are ready for it. No one succeeds without a positive mental attitude, and no one can claim to be mentally fit without it.

In a sense, by developing a positive outlook you are ending an old way of thinking and an old way of living, a way of living without energy and passion in exchange for the exciting adventure, passion, and fulfillment you may long for. Negative thoughts poison the mind and poison the body. Positive thoughts are invigorating and create health. A positive mental attitude is the hallmark of every healthy person.

You can look at it this way. One side of the mind is positive (PMA) and the other side is negative (NMA). Negative thinking cancels out positive thinking, and you can do the math to figure out where that leaves us.

Charles Swindoll, author of teaching materials for home-schooling, presents his perspective on the importance of attitude to set the stage:

The longer I live, the more I realize the impact of attitude on life. Attitude to me is more important than facts. It is more important than the past, than education, than money, than circumstances, than failures, than successes, than what other people think or say or do. It is more important than appearance, giftedness or skill. It will make or break a company, a church, a home. The remarkable thing is we have a choice every day regarding the attitude we will embrace for that day. We cannot change our past. We cannot change the fact that people will act in a certain way. We cannot change the inevitable. The only thing we can do is play on the one string we have, and that is our Attitude. I am convinced that life is 10% what happens to me and 90% how I react to it, and so it is with you. . . . We are in charge of our attitudes.

POSITIVE MENTAL ATTITUDE

We are what we like. All that we are arises with our thoughts.
With our thoughts, we make our world.

—GAUTAMA BUDDHA

Positive Mental Attitude is a combination of three ingredients that Napoleon Hill describes as (1) positive words, such as honesty, faith, love, integrity, hope, optimism, courage, generosity, kindliness, and good common sense; (2) mental powers; and (3) the right attitudes, which are moods or feelings you have toward yourself, another person, a situation, circumstance, or thing. Motivational mottoes such as "Fake it 'til you make it" help temporarily, but they are only sayings, like "Cheer up," which often make people feel worse.

PMA is not an airy-fairy concept—although many people treat it that way. We could call it a positive outlook, positive thinking, an optimistic view, but regardless of what we call it, the foundation for developing and maintaining a positive mental attitude is knowledge and skills or techniques that you are about to learn.

A **positive** attitude is not a destination. It is a **way of life.**

PMA is all about having the mind-set needed to look automatically for the positive in every negative situation. What if you believed that every negative event that happens to you is hiding something positive from you? Something that you will have the good fortune to learn about. Something that will change your life for the better. A place where a gift has been hiding. That's PMA working. There's nothing mystical—it's real. PMA is a healthy way of thinking, it is a way of living and a way of acting and reacting to life's fortunes and misfortunes.

You've heard many times, "Always look for the half-full glass, rather than the half-empty glass." People who think this way jump to look for something positive when things go wrong. People who think this way are not blind or cockeyed optimists. We like to refer to those with PMA as optimists and those with a negative mental attitude (NMA) as pessimists.

We carry within us the resources to do anything we *put our mind to*, from overcoming fears to devising ingenious solutions to the challenges we face. As long as we live we can choose how we will respond to good and bad situations. Building our optimism muscles can be part of an insurance policy, insuring that when adversity knocks, we have the courage to open the door. When opportunity knocks we take advantage of it. So it is with adversity. When adversity knocks, it comes to teach us and it can be a very powerful teacher if we look it square in the face—if we have the right attitude.

> Do all the **good** you can
> By all the **means** you can
> In all the ways **you can**
> In all the places you can
> At **all the times** you can
> To all the people you can
> As long as **you ever can.**
>
> **—JOHN WESLEY**

A positive attitude has the power to change your life. At the present time in human history, fear lurks inside all of us. Many events are out of our control, but there are numerous things we can do to confront fears, make our lives more secure, keep our children safe, do something to feel less vulnerable and taste the joys of life instead of "tackling" . . . "struggling" . . . "surviving" . . . "accepting" what's happening to us.

> It's **never too late** to become what you might have been.
>
> **—GEORGE ELIOT**

Many benefits come with PMA and they are yours for the taking right now. A Positive Mental Attitude . . .

- enables you to think and act constructively.
- helps you to be successful and to fulfill your dreams.
- makes the best of what you have. (You don't spend time worrying about the past or wishing the future would brighten up.)
- encourages you to seize opportunities.
- enhances your ability to control negative thoughts.
- ensures that you have positive thoughts and positive feelings that create a happy life.
- makes every challenge in life a blessing in disguise.

William James (1842–1910), a Harvard Medical School graduate and the founder of psychology as a discipline, firmly believed that life was a battle between pessimism and optimism. He opposed all negative thinking, as he said it fills people with failure and doubt. He believed the universe was full of possibilities. He believed people could improve themselves, improve their lives, and use the mind power within them. He believed that each of us decides our future.

To help you get a deeper understanding of what a positive mental attitude is, how to develop it, and how to reap the many benefits, we are going to explore what the experts have to say about attitude.

WHAT *the* RESEARCH TELLS US *About* ATTITUDE

We're going to arm you with some of the most optimistic research that has inspired us over the years, studies that provide dramatic insights into the benefits of PMA. Then you can *put your mind to it* and go to work on yourself and your attitudes.

The pervasive belief that the mind declines with age is one of the most difficult to erase because it is so deeply embedded in our hearts, minds, and culture. However, we now know, thanks to the pioneering work of Dr. Marian Diamond and others, that the mind, when stimulated and challenged, can continue to learn and grow to the end of life. Indeed, Paul Baltes, a professor of psychology, suggests that we are living in the era of "the continuously developing mind." No longer must we fear the inevitable loss of our mental faculties.

Age can no longer be used as an excuse for not living fully and passionately to the end of life. That, in itself, is one of the most hopeful and optimistic messages of the 21st century. Are you convinced? Isn't that good enough? No, it isn't. Knowing facts that are positive and optimistic won't guarantee that you are optimistic.

There's more. PMA is good for your health. Developing a positive mental attitude that permeates every corner of your life benefits the mind as well as the body. The way this works is via hormones, which have an effect on the immune system. Dr. Christiane Northrup tells us that emotions and thoughts are physically linked to our bodies via our immune, endocrine, and central nervous systems. One of the earliest and most powerful studies of attitude can be found in *Anatomy of an Illness* by Norman Cousins. The author describes how he cured himself from an incurable and life-threatening disease through laughter. His PMA and the effect it had on his immune system literally saved his life.

So we know that PMA is beneficial to health. But that applies only to normal aging, you may say. What about brain diseases? Despite assurances, the specter of Alzheimer's disease lurks in the dark corners of the mind, common responses being fear and anxiety and depression. Some of the most optimistic research on brain disease comes from the now famous Nun Study.

In 1986 Dr. David Snowdon, an epidemiologist, embarked on a revolutionary scientific study of a unique population of 678 Catholic sisters, aged 75 to 106. (This study was mentioned in the Introduction.) By examining the medical histories, cognitive abilities, *and brains* of the nuns of the School Sisters of Notre Dame, Snowdon found dramatic evidence that, while time causes wear and tear on the body, "the mind ages by a unique calendar." Furthermore, the Nun Study provides hope that continued lifelong learning may prevent and/or delay the symptoms of dementia, notably Alzheimer's disease.

> To change your attitude is to change your life.

MORE *on* THE ROLE *of* HOPE

Hope plays a powerful role in life. Far beyond a sunny disposition and a belief that everything will be fine, it means living without the fear of losing our mental faculties, believing that you have the resources to accomplish personal goals and to influence the course of your life. Having hope means believing in a better future. The School Sisters of Notre Dame demonstrate that old age can be a time of promise and renewal, of accepting the lessons that life has taught and passing them on to future generations.

Just as hope has a powerful positive impact on health, a lack of hope may have an equally powerful negative effect. When people learn they have a higher risk of getting Alzheimer's disease, they may conclude that the illness has either already struck—or soon will. And to live in fear of a disease that you don't have and may never develop can serve as a self-fulfilling prophecy.

Snowdon reports on a Mayo Clinic research study in the early 1960s of 839 patients classified as optimists or pessimists on standard personality tests. The study found that 30 years later many more optimists were still alive. Why? The question Snowdon considered was whether the nuns' autobiographies, written when they were healthy young women, could also predict how long they would live.

A careful analysis of 180 autobiographies written when the nuns were young women contained 90,000 words, with 15,298 words relating to emotions. A full 84 percent were positive emotions and only 14 percent were negative. Results showed that emotional content strongly predicted who would live the longest lives—the nuns who used more positive words lived on average 6.9 years longer.

Our mental fitness research identifies a myriad of benefits and tracks significant impacts on individual lives, including improved self-confidence and self-esteem, renewed energy, optimism, and enthusiasm for life. Active engagement in a mental fitness program

> Life is either a **daring adventure** or nothing.
> —HELEN KELLER

contributes to hope, which is one of the most important factors in building and maintaining good health.

While the effect of a mental fitness program in delaying or preventing the onset of Alzheimer's disease may be a contentious issue within academic circles, it isn't for one of our mental fitness participants, Dot Josey, who at the age of 81 claims to be more mentally fit than she has ever been at any other time of her life. And here is what she has to say about it.

"Positive Mental Attitude" by Dot Josey, age 81

I'm one of the fortunate ones who has a PMA. I didn't have to go to university to get it, but I did have to work at it. When I first attended the mental fitness class, I realized I needed to be more positive. I also had to reactivate my learning skills. After much practice "looking on the bright side," my life became happier. I felt motivated, able to cope, to plan and to set achievable goals, and enjoy the satisfaction of seeing them through to completion. It was as though I had been wearing blinkers. Now, I can see the best of every situation and strive for it.

The starting point of all achievements is having a purpose and becoming motivated. As soon as you can name your goal, you can expect many advantages; they come almost automatically. The first advantage is that your subconscious mind begins to work under a universal law. What the mind can conceive and believe, the mind can achieve with a positive mental attitude. When you visualize your goals, your subconscious is affected by the self-suggestions and it goes to work to help get you there.

The second advantage is when you know what you want, there is a tendency for you to get on the right track and head in the right direction. The third advantage of developing a positive mental attitude is that you begin to study, think, and plan. The more you think about your hopes, the more enthusiastic you become, and the more you desire your goal. The fourth advantage—you become alerted to opportunities that help you achieve your goals. When you know what you want, you recognize these opportunities.

A positive attitude keeps you healthier—it gives you a great feeling of well-being. It is a well-known fact that if you have a positive outlook, you will recover more quickly and easily from an illness. I experienced first hand the truth of that seven years ago. I am sure it was my positive attitude that enabled me to be discharged from the hospital less than two weeks after a five-hour bypass heart operation, and return to my volunteer work leading a seniors' fitness class within three months. I learned and grew from that experience. It was my positive attitude that jump-started me to become active again.

Taking part in a mental fitness program has helped me develop an open mind—open to all influences—and it has helped me to develop a curiosity that has spurred me on to learn new things. The program has boosted my self-esteem and made me more confident—but most of all it has inspired me to reach my potential.

Mental abilities do not diminish as we grow older. The challenge is to engage in mental exercise every day in order to cultivate a positive mental attitude. There is no question you will be healthier and happier for it.

Dot Josey was born in England in 1922 and lived in London during the Blitz. She came to Canada as a war bride, raised three sons, and worked most of her married life. Since retirement, she has been a dedicated volunteer at Century House, as a Senior Peer Counselor and a leader of mild physical fitness classes. Dot has been involved in mental fitness from the beginning, providing leadership as Chair of the Lifelong Learning Committee and the Mental Fitness Activity Committee.

ARE YOU *an* OPTIMIST *or a* PESSIMIST?

No explanation of optimism can be complete without reference to the work of Professor Martin Seligman of the University of Pennsylvania, the author of *Learned Optimism*, and the world's leading authority on optimism, helplessness, and explanatory styles. In this chapter we will give you the basics, "Optimism 101." Many of you will want to delve into this subject, and we highly recommend that you do. Dr. Seligman's classic book is a course in itself. To be sure, it will cause provocative discussion and debate and require some of your deepest thinking.

Few people think of themselves as helpless. But the fact is, the main reason people don't succeed is because they do not believe that they can. They have learned to be helpless, a condition that Dr. Seligman calls "learned helplessness," which is the essence of pessimism.

Some people start to believe that they are worthless; they then feel hopeless, which can often lead to anxiety and depression. They stop believing in themselves, in the power of their mind, and they gradually become discouraged. Dr. Seligman calls pessimism a self-fulfilling prophecy and says:

> *Twenty-five years of study have convinced me that if we habitually believe that misfortune is our fault, is enduring, and will undermine everything we do, more of it will befall us than if we believe otherwise. . . . If we are in the grip of this view, we will get depressed easily, we will accomplish less than our potential, and we will even get physically sick more often. Pessimistic prophecies are self-fulfilling.*

According to Dr. Seligman, how you explain life's events determines if you are an optimist or a pessimist. Think about the following three P's (Permanence, Pervasiveness, and Personalization) and how you explain what happens to you.

1. *Permanence*

Pessimists believe that when something bad happens, it will last a long time; they believe the situation or problem is permanent. It's going to last forever. They imagine the worst, are prone to depression, and generally feel helpless. Optimists, on the other hand, believe that bad events or problems are temporary setbacks and have a "this too will pass" atti-

The **measure** of a man is the way he **bears up** under misfortune.

—PLUTARCH

tude. They are not defeated and take the lumps as challenges. They feel in control. How quickly you bounce back from adversity will indicate whether you are an optimist or a pessimist.

2. *Pervasiveness*

Pessimists generalize the problem to their whole life. "It's going to spoil everything." They believe that if they fail in one aspect of their lives, like losing their job, it affects everything; they feel their marriage is, therefore, a failure, and they feel helpless about everything. Dr. Seligman says, "People who give universal explanations for their failures give up on everything when a failure strikes in one area."

> I've never seen a **monument** erected to a pessimist.
>
> —PAUL HARVEY

Optimists explain a bad event as specific to the immediate situation. They may fail in one area, but they don't then feel like failures in life. They may become helpless in one part of their lives, but stay successful and in control of the other aspects. One failure doesn't create total failure.

3. *Personalization*

Pessimists blame themselves. "I'm sorry. It's all my fault." They personalize the problem. Pessimists tend to have low self-esteem and feel worthless and helpless. Optimists think bad events are largely due to external causes. In other words, they don't blame themselves or take things personally.

Some have countered that optimism is merely a sort of false cheerfulness that covers up our real thoughts and feelings. And that these Pollyannas don't take responsibility for anything that happens.

Genuine optimists use the "bad events" or misfortunes as opportunities to improve their lives beyond their wildest—or tamest—dreams. They can search deeply into adversity and turn it into an experience that benefits themselves and often all those near them.

People who have developed a positive mental attitude are not blind optimists. They have learned that in every negative situation there is a gold mine of positives—and the challenge is to dig them out.

HOW *to* BECOME *an* OPTIMIST

The life we live is largely a reflection of our attitudes. And we can change our attitudes by learning a set of skills that help us change the way we talk to ourselves when faced with a setback, misfortune, failure, or any type of adversity. Optimists savor the good things and revel in good times. Dr. Seligman gives us powerful tools that guarantee positive outcomes.

> Problems are only opportunities in work clothes.
> —FREDERICK R. KOPPEL

1. *Dispute your thoughts.*
Launch an attack and argue with your pessimistic thoughts—apply the power thinking you learned in Step 2 to the negative assumptions you may have about your ability to control the events in your life. Change the negative self-talk about your control of the events in your life to a positive attitude.

2. *Teach yourself a lesson.*
Find something positive in a bad situation. Say you are laid off from a job. Figure out what you have lost and then figure out what you have to gain from the experience. Draw a line down the middle of a piece of paper; write losses in one column and gains in the other. Then focus on the gains and on what the experience is trying to teach you.

3. Set realistic goals.

If it's too much to do all at once, do one task per week. Have some fun, take a break and go to a play or movie. Act the way you want to be, and don't spend time around negative people.

4. Think positively.

Focus your mind. Start the day on the lookout for only positive things. In a journal write at least one positive thing that happens every day.

5. Visualize success.

We can change our outlook by playing a movie in our head in which we see ourselves successfully having completed our goals. Real optimists picture themselves accomplishing their goals. They practice visualizing success. They can see the positive results in their mind's eye, and this picture propels them to accomplish what they want.

> Don't stand with your back to the sun and grumble at the shadows.
>
> —ROBERT LOUIS STEVENSON

6. Practice an attitude of gratitude.

Take time to write down all the things you are grateful for. Tell people how grateful you are for such and such. Thank people more and more.

7. Accentuate the positive.

Ask yourself if you are exaggerating a bad situation and blaming yourself. Analyze the situation—what can you do differently? How will a positive attitude help change the situation? Are you over-generalizing? Words like "all-or-nothing" are tips that you are thinking negatively.

More Tips on How to Develop PMA

- Get a change of scenery.
- Do something challenging and fun.
- Do something completely different.
- Break out of your normal routine.
- Create an adventure for yourself and good friends.
- Do something for someone less fortunate than you are.
- Focus on the possibilities.
- Find opportunities in adversity to break free from your old ways of doing things.
- Keep focused on your goals—focused activity reduces procrastination, fear, and anxiety.
- Work on things you enjoy doing.
- Spend time with people who are fun to be around.
- Learn to tell a good joke.
- Laugh out loud when people tell you a joke. Laughter is contagious.
- Work on improving what you do best.
- Don't assume your health will fail.
- Learn to be satisfied with what you have.

> A man can **succeed** at almost **anything** for which he has **unlimited enthusiasm.**
>
> —CHARLES SCHWAB

Now, with a greater awareness of optimism and pessimism, think about your reactions to the information in this chapter and what you might want to change to bring a greater quality of optimism into your life on a daily basis. We invite you to think about the facts concerning how, when, and why to choose a positive mental attitude in everything you do.

PESSIMIST	OPTIMIST
Is always part of the problem	Is always part of the solution
Always has an excuse	Always finds a way to succeed
Says, "That's not my job"	Says, "How can I help you?"
Sees a problem for every answer	Sees an answer for every problem
Thinks it's too difficult	Thinks it's worth a try
Says, "We've never done it before."	Says, "Here's our chance for something new."
Says, "It will never work."	Says, "We'll find a way."
Thinks it's a waste of money	Thinks the investment will be worth it
Says, "We don't have the expertise."	Says, "We'll find an expert."
Thinks it will never work	Believes we can make it work
Thinks it can't be done	Thinks that anything is possible
Thinks it's too radical a change	Is ready for something new
Says, "I don't have any ideas."	Says, "I'll come up with alternatives."
Says, "It's contrary to policy."	Says, "Anything's possible."

This chapter has focused on positive mental attitude. All the components of mental fitness are equally important, yet we introduce them in a logical order, building one upon the other. We won't achieve our goals (Step 1: Goal Setting) if we don't believe we can (Step 2: Power Thinking). If we don't think we are creative (Step 3: Creativity), we won't even try. The only way to achieve a Positive Mental Attitude (Step 4) is through our beliefs (Step 2).

It is essential to have empowering beliefs in order to develop and maintain a positive attitude, and it is essential to have a thorough understanding of PMA before we can incorporate it into our daily lives. Hope begins with power thinking (Step 2), learning to think differently about our beliefs. It is when we change our belief system that we will notice the quality of our lives improve as we change the old messages, the self-talk that disempowers us.

Viktor Frankl's positive attitude did not guarantee his survival in the concentration camps, but he did survive, and he believes one of the reasons was that he used his mind to choose the possibility of survival and thus increased his chances. We do not face the terrors he did, but we can learn from him. By working on a positive mental attitude, we increase our chances of living a healthier and happier life.

In the next chapter, we introduce you to the twin topics of Learning and Memory—two components that are inseparable. But before you begin Step 5, check out the assignment.

ASSIGNMENT

1. For the next 24 hours, talk about everything and every person in a positive way. Then try it for two days. Then three.

2. Start becoming aware of your positive and negative language. Every time you think a pessimistic thought—immediately shift it to a positive one. Try this for seven days and see what happens to your mind when you control it.

3. Set aside five minutes at the end of each day to think some deep, rich thoughts. Write them down in your journal.

4. Optimists express and spread gratitude around. They recognize people for their efforts and give them a pat on the back. Each day give someone a pat on the back—it will build your own optimism muscles.

5. Consider making the "Creed for Optimists" your personal creed.

Creed for Optimists

Be so strong that nothing can disturb your peace of mind.
Talk health, happiness, prosperity to every person you meet.
Make all your friends feel there is something special in them.
Look at the sunny side of everything.
Think only of the best, work only for the best, and expect only
    the best.
Be as enthusiastic about the success of others as you are about
    your own.
Forget the mistakes of the past and press on to the greater
    achievements of the future.
Give everyone a smile.
Spend so much time improving yourself that you have no
    time to criticize others.
Be too big for worry and too noble for anger.

—CHRISTIAN D. LARSEN

STEP

5

MEMORY *and* LEARNING: LEARNING *and* MEMORY

An unused engine rusts. A still stream stagnates.
An untended garden tangles.
It is a powerful and universal truth.

—WALTER M. BORTZ

You have picked up this book for a variety of reasons. You may have jumped right into this chapter because memory is of great interest to you. You don't want to lose it, you want to improve it. You at least want to maintain it—you want to keep the edge. For those of you who started at the beginning, we suspect your memory is already improving and this chapter will tune you up even further. However you approach it, memory is a very important topic. The very fact that you think it is important will serve you well when you *learn what you want to remember*.

There are many good books on the physiology of brain function, how memory actually works in all its scientific complexity. Our approach here is to provide a critical

Turn off the TV—and turn on **your life**.

overview, placing memory squarely with its counterpart, learning.

You may wonder why learning and memory go together. Aren't they very different? Why not deal with them individually? The answer is because learning and memory are inseparable. All the components of mental fitness are interconnected, but the connections between learning and memory are so close that you can't have one without the other. You can't learn anything without engaging your memory, and before you can remember something, you have to learn it. If you can't remember something, it very likely means that you never learned it in the first place.

Why is memory Step 5? The truth is, all the other steps—from goal setting and power thinking to creativity and positive mental attitude—have an impact on learning and memory. We tend to focus too closely on memory to the exclusion of the other components. Now, let's get warmed up. You may be surprised to discover that you actually have an advantage over younger people because you have a lifetime of experience behind you.

♻ WARM-UP

EXERCISE 1

For the first time, we're going to use a Mensa quiz. The reason we have chosen this type of warm-up is to encourage you to try one, to sample another kind of quiz that will stimulate your brain cells and maybe jar your memory. We use Mensa quizzes with our mental fitness classes (adults aged 50 to 94 years) to give their brains a workout. We also experimented one day when we had a group of younger students from the university (aged 25 to 55) join the class. Guess who scored highest? By far the older group scored higher. They had a lifetime of experience and their memory banks held up, whereas many of the younger students had never been exposed to this information. You can't have something in your memory if you haven't put it there. Give this quiz a try:

1. **The fruit of the oak tree A** _____
2. **Which city would you associate with the Reichstag? B** _____
3. **1943 classic film starring Humphrey Bogart and Ingrid Bergman C** _____
4. **She betrayed Samson by cutting off his hair D** _____

5. Creature known as a moose in North America E _____
6. What was the nickname of the American jazz pianist and composer Thomas Wright Waller? F _____
7. What, collectively, were Spike Milligan, Peter Sellers, Harry Secombe, and Michael Bentine? G _____
8. The name in Scotland for New Year's Eve H _____
9. In the USA it is the "Gem State." I _____
10. What word goes before baby, bag, and bean? J _____
11. Where, in Surrey, are the Royal Botanical Gardens? K _____
12. Buddhist monk in Tibet or Mongolia L _____
13. The Roman God of War M _____
14. British Admiral who was in love with Emma, Lady Hamilton N _____
15. Unit of weight, the sixteenth part of a pound O _____
16. Alexandrite, moonstone, and which other gemstone are associated with the month of June? P _____
17. The most powerful piece in chess Q _____
18. Who did the sparrow kill in the nursery rhyme? R _____
19. Whose motto is "Be prepared"? S _____
20. Another name for a tornado in the USA T _____
21. A person in business or insurance who guarantees payment U _____
22. Entertainment art practiced by such performers as Peter Brough, Keith Harris, and Ray Allen V _____
23. In which Belgian town was Napoleon defeated in 1815? W _____
24. What are Finn, Flying Dutchman, and International Tornado classes of? Y _____

To calculate your score, refer to the answers in "Clues and Answers," page 243.

EXERCISE 2: **THE LOST PASSENGER**

Little Billy was four years old and both his parents were dead. His guardian put him on a train to send him to a new home in the country. Billy could neither read nor write nor remember the address, so a large label on a string was secured around his neck clearly indicating Billy's name and destination. However, despite the best efforts and kindness of the railway staff, Billy never arrived at his new home. Why?

EXERCISE 3: **WEATHER FORECAST**

John was watching television. Just after the midnight news there was a weather forecast: "It is raining now and will rain for the next two days. However, in 72 hours it will be bright and sunny." "Wrong again," snorted John. He was correct, but how did he know?

See "Clues and Answers," page 244.

WHAT WE *Have* LEARNED *About* MEMORY

There is a common but false belief that memory loss and aging go hand in hand. Most people believe that they will eventually at some time in their lives not be able to remember things as well as they do now. Forgetting names, forgetting where household items are put, forgetting dates and so on are common events for people of all age groups—however, it creates anxiety in many people as young as 40 who are trying to survive in this fast-paced, high-tech society. They start to convince themselves that it is the beginning of the end.

They may think it is a hopeless situation, instead of thinking about what they can do about it.

There are many reasons for changes in memory that have nothing to do with age or dementia. Some of the common causes are the following:

1. Over-medication or medication interactions
2. Chemical imbalances in the body—not enough potassium, an abnormal thyroid, abnormal blood sugar levels
3. Anxiety and depression or feelings of worthlessness
4. Sudden illness, bacterial infections, flu
5. Chronic illness or disease
6. Malnutrition and dehydration—inadequate diet—not enough fluid in the body
7. Social isolation—living conditions
8. Poverty
9. Decreased sleep
10. Smoking
11. Fatigue
12. Limited vision
13. Limited hearing
14. Inactivity
15. Lack of attention
16. Changes in hormones
17. Boredom
18. Too much alcohol
19. Believing there is nothing you can do for your memory
20. Loss of self-confidence

None of these have anything to do with aging. And there is more good news. This chapter is filled with information on how to reverse the causes of memory loss for people of every age. We aren't minimizing any of these causes nor the commitment that is required to change them. Making healthy lifestyle changes is not easy. Above all, it takes a large dose of self-discipline and determination. However, the results are worth it. In almost every situation—barring diseases of the brain—memory can be improved and the improvement will last a lifetime. This chapter does not deal with diseases; it deals with normal people of all ages and gives you ways to think and act to keep your edge.

Have you ever had this experience? While sitting at your desk, you suddenly realize that you have forgotten a lunch engagement. You begin to feel hot, you get red in the face. Your memory has betrayed you. Are you getting Alzheimer's disease? No. But it's a reminder about something we have all learned: that memory is going to trip us up occasionally.

It is important to realize that no one remembers everything. What we need to know is that we can make decisions every day about what we want to remember and put our efforts into learning those things. No, you are not losing your marbles, although you may wonder where you put them . . .

If you use negative language when referring to your memory—saying things like "My memory's shot" or "I can't remember things the way I used to"—make a conscious effort to stop, and quit worrying. If you want to get down to business, you have to start by shifting to a more positive attitude.

WHAT *Is* MEMORY?

Memory is probably the most well-researched topic in the field of human cognition, which is the academic equivalent of "thinking." Over the years, we have asked many experts a simple question:

"What is memory?" The answer is usually "That all depends." There is *procedural memory*, there is *episodic memory*, and there is *semantic memory*. There is *short-term memory*, there is *long-term memory*, and there is *working memory*. There is also *recall, recollection, recognition,* and *reminiscence.* We want to keep things simple, but it's not easy when research and experience tell us that they aren't.

Although scientists no longer believe in the inevitable decline of memory with age, old assumptions based on that belief continue to discourage many people from keeping their memory in shape. What's old got to do with learning and memory? Absolutely nothing! David Battersby, professor and researcher in the field of Older Adult Education at Massey University in New Zealand, said it best in the following quote:

> *What is meant by aging and being old? The youngest person I know is Elsie, who at 82 has just started her B.A. degree. The oldest person I know is Robert, age 32. He knows everything about everything. He hasn't room for one new idea. His mind is made up. His life is over. So, although he thinks he is quite young, those of us around him know he is very, very old.*

What the Research Tells Us

More than 20 years ago, we attended a seminar presented by a distinguished scholar whose area of expertise was memory. He spoke about memory loss and aging, referring to "young" and "old" subjects, and his message was clear: memory declines as people get older. We said, never mind, what can we do to improve memory as we age? His response was, "You mean, there are ways you can actually improve memory?"

Since that time, scientific understanding of memory has grown: we understand better what it is, and what causes memory loss. So what is memory? One way to understand all that memory encompasses is to think what life would be like if you suddenly lost your memory. We don't just mean that you're suffering from amnesia; imagine you have no memory and no memory capabilities. *Nada.* Zip. Zero. That means

1. You can't reminisce about events or episodes in the past (*episodic memory*)
2. You can't recollect the names of any of the people around you, including your spouse (*semantic memory*)
3. You can't function at all, because you can't remember how to do anything, like driving a car, cooking food, or even opening a door (*procedural memory*)
4. You can't learn anything because you can't remember a thing from one instant to another (*working memory*)
5. You don't know who you are, because the self is a construction of what others think of us and a myriad of events from the time we were born that have shaped who we are

Looking Back to Understand the Present

Let's look more closely, starting with a brief history of memory research. The importance of mental function is clearly reflected in an analysis of findings spanning the past 50 years from the journal *Psychology of Aging and Cognition.* During the 1960s and 1970s, the question most often addressed was whether "the elderly" were capable of functioning at the same level as "younger people." The traditional approach was to view mental function as a general ability that is fixed or "hard-wired" and declines with age; the focus was on tasks that involve learning and memory. Researchers found that older people have lower mental ability than younger people when they tested them in a laboratory setting using a variety of tasks.

Three more recent reviews suggest much of that research was

flawed. Population samples representing "the elderly" ranged from 35 to 100 years of age, and 35, as you would agree, is not old (unless you are a Neanderthal). There were also problems with the methods that were used (for example, labs did not reflect the real world). They suggested age differences could be attributed to flaws in the research design: when speed of response is controlled, differences between young and old can be attributed to the meaningfulness of the task.

> Memory is the treasury and guardian of all things.
>
> —CICERO

In summary, some older people need a little more time to process information because they have such vast stores of knowledge to filter through—furthermore, information must be relevant to them or they won't bother to remember it. When people say their memory is getting worse as they get older, we respond: "Your memory is not getting worse. You just have too much information stored in your brain. If something is important enough, you can make a point to remember it."

Over the past five decades, memory research has become more positive and more practical. Perhaps this reflects the fact that scholars are getting older, and they know it simply isn't true that memory declines with age. They have a personal stake in proving to their much younger colleagues that they aren't "losing it." A more recent research study by Paul Foos and Anna Dickerson is entitled "People

> Memory is the thing I forget with.
>
> —A CHILD'S DEFINITION

My Age Remember These Things Better." Although the memory of older adults is worse in certain areas, they remember other things better than young adults. In other words, at different stages in life, we are involved in different tasks, and we remember particular things that are important to us at that phase and stage of life. It seems logical that we might want to consider the things that older people find important and work on strategies for remembering them. But first, let's take a walk down memory lane.

Memory Lane

Have you ever taken a walk down "memory lane"? These words were coined in 1954 and are defined in Webster's as "an imaginary path through the nostalgically remembered past." We'd like to redefine memory lane. It's a different kind of path, filled with a lifetime of experiences, lessons we've learned the hard way, lessons we've learned the easy way, and the joys that can increase as we age.

For us, this new memory is forward thinking and conjures up a picture of something like Primrose Lane. Remember the old song, "Life's a holiday on Primrose Lane, even roses bloomin' in the lane." It's this optimistic view of memory that we want to imprint on your mind because memory is what we fear losing most. Come and take a walk with us on a new and exciting path down memory lane. It's not always a holiday, but it can be a lot more fun.

> I've never **heard** of an old man (or woman) who forgot where their **money** was hidden.
>
> —CICERO

Webster tells us that memory—derived from the French *memoire*, Latin *mora* (delay), Greek *mermera* (care)—is the power or process of reproducing or recalling what has been learned and retained. The word "remember" means "to bring to mind or think of again; to retain in the memory—for example, the facts until the test is over."

These definitions help us understand the way our memory works: to recollect, recall, recognize, and reminisce mean to bring an image or idea from the past into the mind. To remember implies a keeping in memory that may be effortless or unwilled; to recollect implies a bringing back to mind what is lost or scattered; to recall suggests an effort to bring back to mind and often to re-create in speech; to remind suggests a jogging of memory by an association or similarity; to reminisce implies a casual, often nostalgic recalling of experiences long past and gone.

All this is to say that there are many different aspects of memory—much of it we understand, and much of it we don't. Until recently, almost everything written in the popular literature about memory had an element of doom and gloom. Typically, articles started out something like this:

Use it or lose it. Our memory begins to decline as early as our thirties and forties, but the change is so subtle that we don't notice it. Even if it does not manifest itself, the decline is still going on. And as we age, it takes longer to retrieve information from our memory. We struggle with names, misplace our car keys, forget what we walked into a room for, forget appointments. These are only a few of the things that happen as we age and our memory deteriorates.

That one is pretty blatant. Worse still are the articles that actually tell you what's going to go wrong, sending a message of fear through your whole being. Ironically, these are the messages we can't seem to forget.

We internalize negative images of old age—drawing on common misperceptions and our own experience. On a very deep level, these images cloud our expectations for our own future. Maybe when you were young you visited Granny in a nursing home, sans teeth, sans hair, sans smile. But that's not how it has to be—particularly where memory is concerned.

> We **consider** ourselves as defective in **memory**, either because we **remember** less than we **desire**, or less than we suppose others to **remember**.
>
> —SAMUEL JOHNSON

THE GOOD NEWS *About* MEMORY

The way we talk about and approach the topic of memory is all wrong. You don't become more forgetful as you get older. In fact, you were probably much more forgetful when you were five. That's why, in this book, we are concentrating on how to prevent memory loss by giving you strategies to keep your mind challenged and stimulated, strategies for developing an excellent memory for the things that matter most to you. And we are going to use everything we know to empower you, to give you hope and optimism for a brighter and more memorable future.

You are in control of your mind, no one else is, and you can, with some effort, keep your memory functioning until the day you die. You can improve your memory as you age, as well as ward off specific concerns. You may also be able to prevent or delay the onset of diseases such as Alzheimer's.

The Case of the Lost Mittens

Do you remember the string on your mittens, going from one mitten, up through one arm of your parka, and down the other arm to the other mitten? Why? Because five-year-olds don't remember where they leave their mittens. Not because their brains aren't working or haven't developed, but because they're having too much fun and they aren't paying attention. They're not concentrating— the same reason we forget our gloves when we're 95 years old.

- How is it that a 16-year-old forgets to be home by midnight?
- How is it that a 19-year-old forgets her driver's license?
- How is it that a 27-year-old forgets his wedding anniversary?
- How is it that a 46-year-old forgets what she went upstairs for?
- And how is it that a 95-year-old can remember to show up for bridge on time?

Despite what you read or what you may think, memory problems in later life are not very different from what we experienced in our youth. We just worry about it more—and worry and anxiety are major causes of memory loss at any age.

As far as general physiology is concerned, memory is too often written about in terms of loss and decline, even though some writers are careful to explain that decline is not as precipitous as previous studies indicated. Nonetheless, they tell us that very few people avoid deteriorating memory, and it's the exception rather than the rule that people in their 80s and 90s can still "play with a full deck." They tell us that basic physiological changes continue throughout life, including cell loss, poorer connections between neurons, and lower levels of chemicals (neurotransmitters). Add up all the cognitive changes, and you've got an old brain that simply isn't firing on all cylinders. Comedians refer to "senior moments," and they get a lot of laughs. But humor is sadly misplaced when it reinforces negative stereotypes about aging.

> A memory without blot or contamination must be an exquisite treasure, an inexhaustible source of pure refreshment.
>
> —CHARLOTTE BRONTË

It is true that our bodies and our minds and our spirits change as we age. There is no question we get more wrinkles. There is no question our spirits can be enriched in later life. There is also no question that our minds can stay powerful—and become even more powerful—as we age.

Many writers talk about "normal memory loss." However, *dementia is a disease.* Memory loss that occurs with dementia of any kind is not a part of normal aging. (We used to say, "Mother's going senile," which means she's "losing her marbles.") A small percentage of older adults suffer from dementia; however, we don't deal with dementia in this book, with the exception of references to breakthroughs in research.

What most people want to know is how to recognize early signs of dementia. Most of us may forget the name of a person we just met but not that we just met someone. (After you learn to use the techniques in this chapter, you will remember the names of those you choose to remember.) It is normal to forget where you put your car keys, but not what the keys are for. (Once you master the techniques in this chapter, you will always remember where your car keys are.) It is normal to repeat a story to someone but not normal to constantly repeat the same story or ask the same question. And it is not normal to forget your own date of birth. If, however, you keep telling people you are 39 and holding, you may start to confuse yourself and your year of birth. And once you are over 80—a ripe age beyond maturity—you may find that you begin to add years. Not because you have forgotten how old you are, but because you are proud of how you feel and look and want to impress people with how old you are.

TAKING CHARGE *of* YOUR MEMORY

People can remember anything they *have a mind to*. Listen carefully to what people around you say about their memory, forgetting, and learning; and listen to yourself. You'll be amazed at the derogatory things people say. We blame a lot on aging, but it's not the culprit. If you take the time to study the material in this chapter, it will have a positive effect on the quality of your life for the rest of your life. You won't ever need to use aging as an excuse. It will be a challenge—but it's these very challenges we set for ourselves and work on that create healthy brains, which serve us . . . forever.

You've got a lot to lose by not taking up the challenge—and everything to win if you take it up. The odds are completely in your favor. You can even make a game out of learning and incorporating the following strategies into your everyday life. It's worked for countless others, and it can work for you.

There are numerous strategies that can assist us in never having to worry about remembering again. We will outline the things people say they have trouble with and offer practical ways to rectify them. Not everyone says they have trouble remembering these things—and you might not. After you've finished, take note of areas that you will want to improve and then read on. It's when you start remembering to learn that your mind will improve. Your brain will love it, and so will you.

In this section, you will learn about the most common items that people say they have trouble remembering. Most often when people have trouble remembering, it is because they have not learned it well enough in the first place. When we learn something, we have placed it in our minds so that it is stored and ready for use. If we don't remember it, chances are very good we didn't learn it in the first place.

For each of the items most commonly forgotten, we give you a strategy. Learn and practice these and, if you do, you will begin to see enormous change. You will be in control of your mind, how and what you put into it, and you will reap the good feelings that come with remembering what you want to.

There is no parking lot for employees where I work, so each day I drive around the block and park my car on a nearby side street. At the end of the day, I walk out of the building and wander around looking for my car. It's not that I can't remember where it is—I didn't learn where I left it. I didn't make a "mental note" of which street I parked on or how far up the block or in front of which store. I didn't

Memory is a capricious and arbitrary creature. You never can tell what pebble she will pick up from the shore of life to keep among her treasures, or what inconspicuous flower of the field she will preserve as the symbol of "thoughts that do often lie too deep for tears" . . . and yet I do not doubt that the most important things are always the best remembered.

—HENRY VAN DYKE

pay attention, observe, or learn. If I had done those things, I would remember exactly where I parked my car. Most days, it really doesn't matter and I don't mind wandering around a bit. I've noticed, however, that if I have a meeting scheduled after work, I always pay attention to where I park, and later in the day, I can locate the car quickly.

The best strategy is to take careful note of where you park. If you're in a parking garage, check the level (2B, for example) and the north–south orientation, and make up something that will fix it in your mind, like "Shakespeare didn't go north to Alaska, but he said, 'To be or not to be,' and in this case it is 2B." It can be great fun creating your own "location code"—it exercises your mind in a positive way and you will remember where you parked your car.

THE "TIP of the TONGUE" EXPERIENCE

Gloria Levi and Kathy Gose, in their book *Dealing with Memory Changes as We Grow Older*, tell us that the human brain contains tremendous amounts of information, some of which cannot be tapped and retrieved at any given moment. Although you know the information is stored, you may feel as though you are looking for a needle in a haystack. You know it's there, but you cannot put your finger on it.

When you are having difficulty recalling the name of someone you know, you are having a "tip of the tongue" experience. You may be able to picture the person in your mind's eye, or remember some part of his or her name or a name like it, or the rhythm or general sound of the name. Or you can remember other information about the person, such as where you met. You are almost able to recall the name, but not quite. Finally, you say, "It's on the tip of my tongue" because you know you have the knowledge stored. You are trying all your clues and associations, but you still cannot retrieve it.

An internal monitor appears to operate as you search the pathways of associations to the information you are seeking. This monitor seems to say, "Go and retrieve. If you do not find what you are looking for down one pathway, try another and another, until you do find it."

The search might go something like this: "Now what is the name of that woman with the curly hair who is Susan's friend? I think her name begins with R, or is it B? Rooster? No, that couldn't be it—Brewster? Yes, that's it! And her first name, is it biblical?—Sarah, Rebecca, Judith? No, none of these. Elizabeth, Martha, Mary? I'm getting close. It's Mary something. Mary Anne, Mary Elizabeth? Oh wait, it's the same as my granddaughter's—Rosemary. No, not quite, but it does have a flower in it. Ah, it's Mary Rose—Mary Rose Brewster. At last!"

The monitor will recognize what you are looking for and will discard information that doesn't fit. However, from time to time it may get stuck on a word that closely resembles the one you are seeking. For example, the name you want is "Mary Rose" but the one that keeps popping up in your head is "Rosemary," your granddaughter's name. You may have difficulty retrieving "Mary Rose" because it is blocked by "Rosemary."

But the monitor will continue working on an unconscious level long after you have given up trying, and often the correct name will suddenly appear. You might wake in the middle of the night remembering a name you have been looking for earlier that day. Everyone has experienced the delight and sense of relief when, after a long search, the information you are seeking seems to pop into your head.

The tip of the tongue experience suggests that something you are looking for in long-term memory is not where you expected it to be. The name you want is organized and stored in many ways, surrounded by a web of associations. To retrieve it you will need to find the associations that will lead you to the name itself.

The fact that you have been circling around the name, picking up different clues that tell you something about it, indicates that people remember information in pieces. Though you often remember only part of something, through a series of clues you can reach more and more of what has been stored. Key words, sights, smells, sounds, tastes are all clues.

The next time you have a tip of the tongue experience, give yourself a few moments to go through the clues you used to recall the information you were seeking. Not only is this pleasant and reassuring, it helps to anchor the information in your memory more securely.

Most people feel embarrassed when they can't remember someone's name. They think they are losing their memory. They feel stupid. These feelings set up a huge block for the mind to recall the name. There will be times when you forget a name, but there are two ways of dealing with it that will change the process forever in your life.

The first thing is to realize you are not losing it. You are not remembering for a whole variety of reasons addressed in this chapter—few, if any, have to do with aging, and most we can control. The second thing is to realize that you probably have not learned the name sufficiently well. To address the first issue, we need to develop an approach to take if, on occasion, you don't recall someone's name. First of all, don't say, "I'm sorry, I can't remember your name." Say something like "Your name is on the tip of my tongue." If the person is offended and says something like "You don't remember my name? It's Mary Ann, and we've known each other for four years!" Your job is to turn these negatives into positives (Step 4). Say something like this: "It's not my memory, Mary Ann. I had a very poor sleep last night and I'm very tired."

SIX MOST COMMON THINGS PEOPLE WANT *to* REMEMBER

A study by Von Leirer and colleagues at Stanford University asked which memory skills people would most like to improve. In order of importance, they are:

1. People's names
2. Important dates and appointments
3. Location of household items
4. Recent and past events
5. When to take vitamins and medications
6. Important information and facts

For confirmation, we asked the members of a mental fitness class to tell us what they would like to learn and/or improve. Their responses were consistent with the test scores, with 1 being the most common challenge and 6 being the least. Before we go any further, you are invited to test yourself on common memory challenges.

The following is a list of the common memory challenges that people of all ages experience. How often does this happen to you? Score yourself from 1 to 5 according to the following 5-point scale. The higher the score, the better your memory function.

1 — never

2 — seldom

3 — sometimes

4 — frequently

5 — always

I _____ remember people's names.

I _____ remember important dates.

I _____ remember the location of household items.

I _____ remember recent and past events.

I _____ remember to take vitamins and medications.

I _____ remember important information and facts.

Learning People's Names

When you meet people for the first time, alert your brain to the upcoming challenge. Instead of saying to yourself something like "Omigod, I'm not good at remembering names" or "I'll never remember his name," say to yourself, "Here's my chance to give my brain a workout. I'm going to relax, take a deep breath." Think positively, know that you can and will learn his name. Then pay close attention to the name, repeat it as you are introduced, and don't shy away from names that are difficult to pronounce. If you don't hear it, ask for it to be repeated. Make a game out of learning it and don't hurry. It could go something like this:

"Bill, I'd like you to meet Victoria Moore. We play bridge together. Victoria, this is Bill Atchou."

"Nice to meet you, Victoria. I used to play bridge years ago."

"Did you, Bill? I missed how to pronounce your last name."

"Oh, it's Atchou, just like when you sneeze—you know—Atchou!"

"Bless you, Bill."

And so it goes, back and forth, using the person's name as many times as possible in the first minute or two of introductions. It's a great technique for embedding the name in your brain. Saying "How do you do, Victoria," once is usually not enough for the brain to learn the name. The more you use this technique, the better you'll get, and then you can teach it to others. It works, it's fun, and you'll be surprised how good you will feel. The next time you see Bill, you can give him a tissue.

> My mind lets go of a thousand things,
> Like dates of wars and deaths of kings,
> And yet recalls the very hour—
> 'Twas noon by yonder village tower,
> And on the last blue moon in May—
> The wind came briskly up this way,
> Crisping the brook beside the road;
> Then, pausing here, set down its load
> Of pine-scents, and shook listlessly
> Two petals from that wild-rose tree.
>
> —THOMAS BAILEY ALDRICH

Here's another technique: associate the name with something familiar or funny. Perhaps the place you met is unusual. Pay attention to where you meet someone. This association will help your learning process, too. Remember where you met Ramona? Your children and grandchildren won't, because they never learned that song. "Ramona, we'll meet beside the waterfall."

Remembering Important Dates and Appointments

Being organized is important when it comes to remembering. The trick here is not having to remember. No one at any age remembers all the appointments and things they have to do. While it may be a good mental workout to memorize a list of daily tasks, there is a better way. Make a habit of writing down the important dates and things you want to do on a calendar, in a daily journal, or on a pocket computer—whatever works best for you (*not* little scraps of paper).

Make lists, write things down, and develop good habits to assist your memory. Do things at the same time each day—for example, review tomorrow's schedule of events the evening before and *then* check it over during your morning routine. Don't pack your day so full that you don't have time to think clearly. Plan your meetings and your errands so you can avoid peak hours in traffic.

Write down all the things you want to do. Write down as much as you need to. Keep notebooks, notepads, and pens or a pocket computer available and jot down things when they pop up in your mind. You might want to have notebooks in certain rooms or in your purse. Developing the habit of writing things down is a good way to capture your thoughts—the very act of writing is a form of mental rehearsal that assists your memory.

Being organized is important when it comes to remembering. Each person can devise effective strategies that foolproof the mind. Organizing, developing habits, and creating your own strategies work. Here are some tried and true methods—use them as they are, adapt them to your needs, or create your own unique strategies. These may seem obvious, but not everyone uses them. Keep a calendar in the same spot for important dates and appointments. If you use a pocket or purse calendar and one on your kitchen wall, then you must check them both each day— or transfer one to the other.

A Place for Everything and Everything in Its Place

Design an area in your home, perhaps in your home office, that has a table or desk with all your memory tools: a calendar, bulletin board, place to store bills, glasses (keys hang on a special hook near your front door). The calendar can be used for important dates—to pay bills, or important events, doctor's appointments, exercise.

You might want to consider having two calendars—kept in the same place—one for important business dates, volunteer work, and doctor's appointments, and one for social events and other engagements. This is another area where you can experiment until you find the strategies that work for you. Get creative—see Step 3. It's good for your brain to figure out what it needs that will work in your situation. And send us the hard ones you have managed to conquer and we'll share them.

Remembering Where You Put Important Household Items

Have one place in your home where you hang your keys. As soon as you are home hang them there. Make a habit of it. If you are out anywhere, at someone's house, for instance, put your keys in a special compartment in your purse or in your pants pocket—make a habit of it. Stop using aging as an excuse for not finding your keys. Your mind will cooperate if you do, and you'll always know where your keys are.

Use the same strategy for all household items. Have a special drawer for scissors, tape, etc.—and always put them right back after you use them. Can you hear your mother saying, "Remember to put them back right where you found them!" and "A place for everything and everything in its place."

Your mother probably also said, "An ounce of prevention is worth a pound of cure." Organizing your items is the prevention. However, if you don't put them back where they belong right away and can't find them, it's better to go and buy a new pair than to fuss and fume for an hour trying to find them and calling yourself names under your breath. This kind of stress is bad for your health, and it isn't worth the $6 you'll spend on new scissors. Besides, by the time you get back from the store, you will likely walk into your house and they'll be sitting somewhere in plain view—right where you left them. But remember, one in the hand is worth two in the drawer. Next time you need scissors, you'll have two in your hand. So the message is . . . decide to have some fun with your memory. Play some tricks on it—and it won't be so inclined to play tricks on you.

> The secret of a good memory is attention, and attention to a sub-ject depends upon our interest in it. We rarely forget that which has made a deep impres-sion on our minds.
>
> —TYRONE EDWARDS

Remembering Recent and Past Events

In the following situations, which of the names do you think you might remember? Rank them in order of importance to you, number 1 being most important, number 5 being least important. What does this tell you about remembering events?

1. The name of someone who owes you $50
2. The name of someone who works with your neighbor
3. The name of someone to whom you owe $1.50
4. The name of someone who brought regards from your nephew
5. The name of someone who borrowed a book from you

Remembering to Take Vitamins and Medications

Once again, organization is the key, and putting out your medications in the evening works well. There are many different kinds of containers to use—daily, weekly, or monthly—that you can pick up at the drugstore. Here, too, you can get creative and make your own. Use simple egg cartons or labeled containers for each day of the week, some marked a.m. and some p.m.

If you take medications when you are away from home, develop a method for remembering when to take them. For example, make up a jingle for coffee time—when you take your first sip of coffee, make up a rhyme such as: "Coffee time is Fem-time [a type of vitamin]." In fact, creating a riddle or jingle is good mental exercise and helps you take control of your memory. It also helps you to lighten up—and any way that you can reduce stress will help your memory. Routine is very important.

Remembering Important Information and Facts

Of the six most common memory challenges, this is the one that most closely reflects the process of learning in the way that we typically think of learning—that is, in relation to education.

Many people have played themselves to death, or eaten and drunk themselves to death. Nobody has ever thought himself to death. The chief danger confronting us is not age. It is laziness, sloth, routine, stupidity—many who avoid learning find that life is drained dry. But no learner has ever run short of subjects to explore. The pleasures of learning are indeed pleasures.

"The key to a good memory is interest," claims Dr. Bruce Whittlesea, a psychology professor from Simon Fraser University who has been studying memory and teaching memory techniques for the past 20 years. Ever forget a face, or an anniversary, or where you parked? Chances are you failed to make a mental note. People tend to blame forgetfulness on a bad memory, but that's not the case. You remember things best when you're interested. It's really a decision we make at the outset, whether something is worth the trouble to remember. Most people misunderstand memory. People tend to think that remembering is all memory does. In fact, that's its least important function. How people code the information in their environments has everything to do with how they function. People think, "The world is there; you pick it up," but that's wrong. What people really do is reinvent and reconstruct the world for themselves, every moment of every day.

In *The Mind Map Book*, Barry and Tony Buzan introduce a particular strategy for reconstructing learning and memory. The tool is the mind map, and it works both for taking notes quickly and efficiently and for remembering a large amount of information at a glance. Sandra used it in her doctoral studies, and you can use it in every area of life if it works for you. We highly recommend it because

1. It is a quick and efficient method for note-taking at a lecture or presentation.
2. It uses your unique creativity—no two mind maps are ever the same.
3. It simulates graphically what is going on in your brain cells (neurons) as the dendrites branch out and develop new connections.
4. It can be used as both a way of learning and a way of remembering a large amount of information at a glance.

The news that comes to us at the beginning of the 21st century is cause for great celebration. Results of current research on the lifelong development of the mind are extremely optimistic and hopeful. Indeed, Paul Baltes refers to the 21st century as the "era of the continuously developing mind." Research by noted scholars such as Marian Diamond, Arne Scheibel, and Paul Nussbaum tells us we can continue to learn and grow for as long as we live. And the longer we learn, the healthier we become.

The pioneering work by Marian Diamond demonstrates that mental stimulation alone, regardless of age, can have a direct and significant effect on the immune system; the pathway is via hormones that are released under stress. The possibility of improving one's own immune system by stimulating and challenging the brain is revolutionary. In a study in the 1980s, playing bridge improved the immune system— and we believe that your personal mental fitness program can have the same effect.

We know that physical exercise improves mental and emotional health; however, many frail elderly people cannot participate in physical exercise due to disabilities and diseases. Believe it or not, we now know that mental activity alone can benefit physical health. Social activities that require less physical exercise, such as learning something new, may complement physical exercise programs, particularly for frail elderly persons. Which means that learning has health benefits for everyone.

Paul Nussbaum's research is leading the way in the growing understanding of learning as a health-promoting behavior. The brain requires stimulation and challenge at every age. Learning is vital for overall health and brain wellness, and it should be regarded as a standard part of any existing health program. Furthermore, Nussbaum suggests that learning can serve as a vaccination against

You can take all the wonder pills and use all the creams that promise to alter the course of aging, and if they work at all, their effects will pale compared to that of a single continuing education course that stimulates your thinking and motivates you to try something new and interesting.

—GENE COHEN

late-life neurodegenerative diseases of the brain. Much research is aimed at slowing and possibly curing brain diseases. Now, we are starting to focus on lifestyle behaviors, such as learning, that might reduce the risk of developing Alzheimer's disease.

Studies have confirmed that learning new things causes dendrites to grow and branch wildly, improving your brain power. We now know that the most benefits come from learning about something that is quite different from what you have learned in the past. If you have always wanted to take piano lessons, for example, now is the time. Learning a new language has also been shown to have great benefit.

Your ability to learn is affected by a healthy lifestyle. Physical fitness, good eating habits, and so on all make a difference to learning. As well, limiting beliefs are often below our level of awareness. Any strategies that create heightened awareness of limiting beliefs is a start. Once they are identified, they have to be replaced with positive beliefs.

Everybody has a particular learning style—certain ways of learning that work best for that particular individual. For example, some people like to learn by doing, others prefer to listen to an expert. Some people prefer to learn independently, by taking correspondence courses or courses online and reading. However, we know that there is one tried and true method that works for everyone—and that is group discussion and dialogue. Take a risk—accept a challenge—and jump in with both feet. We don't know of anyone who was ever sorry they did.

Start believing that you can improve your memory and learn anything you choose. Concentrate hard on whatever you want to learn, create a mental picture of what you want to remember. Ask people to speak up and repeat anything you don't hear, and cultivate an attitude of fun. Repeat and review things you want to remember, eliminate any form of anxiety and stress, and constantly challenge yourself to learn new things.

Learning is one of the pleasures of life. It is not confined to book learning, academics, or school. Learning means keeping an open mind, one that is willing to receive all new things, one that wants to create and change and grow. Learning extends our lives in new dimensions and new directions. Never stop learning, no matter what age you are. Every age and every phase of life present new opportunities to learn.

- I've learned that if you spread the peas out on your plate, it looks like you ate more.—age 6
- I've learned that the great challenge of life is to decide what's important and disregard everything else.—age 51
- I've learned that enthusiasm is caught, not taught.—age 51
- I've learned that life sometimes gives you a second chance.—age 62
- I've learned that people are as happy as they decide to be.—age 79
- I've learned that when I eat fish sticks, they help me swim faster, because they're fish.—age 7

STEP

SPEAKING
Your MIND

*We look forward to a world founded upon four essential human
freedoms. The first is the freedom of speech and expression.*

—Franklin D. Roosevelt

N ot everyone wants to climb on a soapbox and address the crowd. There are many forms of expression and forums for speaking your mind. We present a variety of communication modes, making distinctions between conversation, discussion, debate, and dialogue. We'll explore the revival of two traditions that you may want to join or start in your community: the philosopher's café and the conversational salon. Finally, we'll give you some instructions regarding how to start your very own salon and how to ensure that it is successful. The Oxford Dictionary defines communication as "being in touch by words or signals, using all kinds of methods to make people understand." But first, it's time for a warm-up exercise.

WARM-UP

EXERCISE: THE MAN IN THE PAINTING

A man stands in front of a painting and says the following: "Brothers and sisters have I none. But this man's father is my father's son." How is the man in the painting related to the man who is in front of it? (See "Clues and Answers," page 244.)

MEDIATED COMMUNICATION

Before we begin our discussion of different forms of face-to-face communication between people, it's important to consider how many ways there are of communicating that do not require people being together—like this text. In today's high-tech world, mediated communication influences our working, public, and private lives to an astounding degree, and we often have little information about the source, the reliability, or the validity of the message. The journalist Allen Garr writes about communication as an illusion that supports and encourages dishonesty. According to Garr, "What is variously called the electronic age, the digital age or the age of virtual reality has turned us into a culture of fabricators and fibbers. The human element has been removed from the communications equation and replaced by illusion. As Gertrude Stein once said, 'There is no there there.'"

Have you ever . . .

- spent 30 minutes pushing buttons on your telephone to get the information you want and suddenly have the line go dead?
- phoned someone who "screened you out" and didn't pick up the phone?
- rehearsed the message you want to convey, or written it down, only to be tongue-tied when your call was answered by a human being?
- told a friend not to answer the phone so that you can leave a message?

INTERFACING FACE-*to*-FACE

All this technology creates a virtual reality, leaving people hungry for old-fashioned methods of communication with breathing, thinking, caring human beings. The lost art of conversation is currently experiencing a revival. Conversation is defined in one dictionary as "good talk practiced as an art" and may take the form of discussion, which simply refers to "verbal exchange of ideas"; or debate, which means to "discuss thoroughly as in a formal discussion under certain rules of procedure."

This chapter is not a mini-course in public speaking. There are numerous good books and programs for that. We offer an opportunity to consider the various venues for you to speak your mind, anything from a welcome speech at a family reunion to a eulogy at a close friend's funeral, and everything in between. It is your opportunity to change the world with words. We need only think of some of the great people and phrases we associate with them to realize how much impact speaking has. To name a few, Martin Luther King's "I have a dream"; John F. Kennedy's "Ask not what your country can do for you, ask what you can do for your country"; Winston Churchill's "We shall fight them on the beaches . . . we shall never surrender." These words changed the world. They changed your world, they changed our world. Theodore Roosevelt liked to quote the old adage "Speak softly and carry a big stick; you will go far." In your own world your words can add joy to a celebration, they can have a positive impact in your child's schoolyard, they can inspire a friend, or they can land you a job.

WHY SPEAK *Your* MIND?

Speaking your mind is so important that doing it can change how you feel about yourself. Every day in every way, speaking your mind builds confidence and a sense of joy in life. It helps us face problems by articulating our feelings. Asserting yourself in a positive way is a key part of speaking your mind. There are many assertiveness training courses available—the ones with excellent facilitators are worth their weight in gold.

There is nothing that feels quite as good as expressing your deepest thoughts concerning something of meaning and value to you, knowing that people are listening and that they understand exactly what you are saying and how you feel. This last component of mental fitness will help you gather those thoughts and unleash them on the world in just the right place at the right time for maximum impact.

Speaking your mind is a key component of mental fitness for many reasons. The first is obvious. It's satisfying to think clearly, critically, and creatively, but if you don't speak your mind, you cannot engage the world. If you are mentally fit, you have "a good head on your shoulders," and if you have lived for 40, 50, or 100 years, you have learned and experienced things that other people need and want to hear about. You have a perspective on the important things in life that is supported by well-tested beliefs and values.

> My best friend is the person who brings out the best in me.
>
> —HENRY FORD

This brings us to the second reason why speaking your mind is so critical. You may have been trained since childhood to respect authority and to keep your mouth shut. If so, you may have to overcome a lifetime of training that began with "Children should be

seen and not heard." If you are a woman over 50, you have probably learned your lessons all too well, and it may take time and commitment to unlearn them. If you were born between 1946 and
1961, you are considered part of the baby boom generation. These
dates vary from study to study, but it is generally accepted that this
15-year postwar period makes up the baby boomers. Think about
the term "boomer"—it came about because of the demographic
swell, the huge increase in births between 1946 and 1961. There are
75 million baby boomers in North America. If the boomers were to
speak their minds, what a boom it would make!

Generally speaking, baby boomers are interested in strategies
such as exercise, diet, and mental fitness to promote a healthy, long
life. This demographic group is large and diverse: the older
boomers are refusing to grow older—and using whatever means
there are to maintain their youth. The younger boomers, now in
their early 40s, have learned the hard way that it's important to
speak your mind; they are also the very first group to have an optimistic view of aging.

We want you to read and think about something new, both personally and professionally. We invite you to consider different views
and different venues for all kinds of communication. Try out new
ways to speak your mind—and to change the world if you choose to
or, even more important, to change yourself. And if you don't really feel like changing the world or yourself, then take a well-deserved
break and just for fun, read about the philosopher's cafés and
salons of another era, which are making a comeback.

A large portion of the older population today are part of what
Ann Fishman, president of Generational-Targeted Marketing,
calls "the Silent Generation." As many as a third of the population
over 50 are part of that generation. If we consider that a third of
the total population in North America is over 50, we are talking

about 11 percent of the total population—as many as 40 million people in the United States alone.

The Silent Generation, born between 1925 and 1942, is the generation either currently retiring or recently retired. They make up the population roughly between 60 and 80 years old who are today's pioneers in redefining what it means to be "older" in an aging world. They are generally vital and active people—exploring new opportunities and adventures. Within this group are the great feminists and civil rights advocates whose mission in life has been to "humanize the world." They have high principles, respect for experts, and a strong work ethic, and are generally motivated by a willingness to be helpful to others. But many in this generation are silent, only rarely making their voices heard.

> We confide in our strengths, without boasting of it; we respect that of others, without fearing it.
>
> —THOMAS JEFFERSON

Many, particularly the women, make their greatest contributions through the family—as daughters, wives, mothers, and grandmothers. In deferring to authority, however, they may fail to make their voices heard in the wider community. But things are changing now: these people have more opportunities than ever before and are taking advantage of them. Many community programs present a forum for people to practice their speaking skills, to explore their passions, and thus to emerge from the voiceless closet.

A group of us from the Mental Fitness for Life program, comprising people aged 50 to 85, took our mental fitness message to the World Congress on Aging in 2001 in Vancouver, where delegates from 65 countries had gathered. We presented perspectives on the mental fitness program, and 300 delegates—researchers, scholars, and practitioners—were there to listen.

CONVERSATIONAL SKILLS

The ability to speak effectively can be learned by anyone and is an invaluable asset in all aspects of our lives—personal, professional, social, and volunteer. It is important for well-being, self-confidence, and self-esteem. There is a great deal of personal satisfaction in being able to present ideas clearly and concisely. And, really, when you think about it, conversation is a way that you can enjoy yourself and help others to enjoy themselves.

Speaking your mind is a powerful tool for people of all ages. It affords numerous opportunities in your personal and work life, whether you are talking from your seat in a friendly conversation or from your feet to a group of colleagues. You will have pride in yourself and be considered a leader in your professional and volunteer work.

Speaking effectively is an art. It is an excellent way to train your mind and to cultivate a vocabulary and expressive style that is truly yours. Giving voice to your thoughts, expressing what you really want to say, being courageous, being kind, are all hallmarks of a healthy mind.

Seize every opportunity for speaking your mind—it gives your brain cells a good workout. Think before you speak—what is it that you really want to say? Join in discussions—everyone has something important to contribute. Don't talk to people or at people or over their heads. Talk *with* people and then, above all, listen. Wendy's father always used to say, "Don't use a 25-cent word when a 5-cent one will do," and Thomas Jefferson used to say, "The most valuable of talents is that of never using two words when one will do."

We all grow up using language, but few people today have an appreciation and understanding of conversation. If we receive any education at all in public speaking, it is training in the art of debate. We are taught how to use words strategically to attack an opponent's weak points, to defend our opinions, to cut our opponent to shreds with a few sharp words, to shoot down someone else's ideas and to demolish their arguments. This is clearly not conversation but a very civilized form of warfare.

Suppose we began conversations not to persuade others, but to learn about them? Imagine how different life would be if, instead of competing in conversation, we were taught to value speaking itself. Suppose we approached conversation aesthetically: What if we began to look for elegance, beauty, and simplicity; to appreciate charismatic and creative delivery; to become engaged and transported by words? Suppose we listened to discover the complex beauty of another person's ideas instead of listening with the intent of finding flaws? We might become wiser and more eloquent.

THE ART *of* CONVERSATION

According to David Battersby, a pioneer in Third Age learning, it is the need for and the emphasis on discussion and dialogue that distinguish mature adult learners from adult learners in general. Furthermore, in a skillfully facilitated or moderated adult learning class, the roles of teacher and learner are interchangeable. The facilitator's primary role is to provide a comfortable context and climate within which people engage freely and passionately in discussion about matters of personal interest or concern. The emphasis is on discussion that is liberating and empowering, that puts people fully in charge of their own thoughts and feelings.

Through discussion, people develop their own ideas more fully and come to understand different points of view. Through discussion that is based on mutual respect and a genuine interest in what others have to say, people gain greater respect for themselves. In addition to a willingness and a desire to express one's own beliefs, values, and opinions, one must also be a "good listener." How many people do you know who like to monopolize conversations but don't seem to be really interested in what you have to say?

When someone is truly interested in your point of view, it is a gift. Listen with your ears, your heart, and your mind. When someone is presenting an idea, you don't need to be gathering your thoughts for a response, or looking for an argument to prove you are right. You don't need to be threatened by some-

A drop of honey catches more flies than a gallon of gall.

one else's knowledge, and you don't need to fear that you will not sound intelligent. Just listen, take it in, relax. Maybe all you need to do is ask a few questions—never mind your own story. Consider what you could learn from the other person's point of view. What is he or she really trying to tell you? Give them the gift of true listening, and you will see them glow. Then, on a different day, at a different time, speak your mind and seek out someone who will do the same for you.

DISCUSSION *and* DIALOGUE

A discussion group brings people together to process new information, reinterpreting it in the context of life experience. How do you know when you have had a successful discussion? Is it because people think you are brilliant? Is it because everybody was listening? Quite simply, you will feel good—more specifically and more importantly, you will have more energy. And what could possibly be a greater gift than the gift of life-giving energy? When people give each other energy, exciting things happen.

At the present time, there is a great need to go beyond discussion to a much deeper form of communication so that people from different cultures and countries can live together harmoniously. According to Daniel Yankelovich, communications advisor to corporations, government, and professional organizations in the United States, now more than ever there is a need for real dialogue in business settings. The need to dialogue comes as a result of many factors, such as the following:

- the steady erosion of authority in the workplace
- the trend toward alliances between organizations that bring different cultures, structures, and traditions to new partnerships
- the need to repair the damage to morale that results from downsizing
- the need to stimulate creativity and innovation

Webster defines dialogue as seeking mutual understanding and harmony. However, the outcome of every conversation is not always harmonious. It may be enough that people come to understand why they disagree so vehemently. Martin Buber, in his masterpiece, *I and Thou*, suggests dialogue implies a genuine openness to each other. I do not selectively tune out the view with which I disagree nor do I marshal arguments to rebut—rather I take in the other's viewpoint, engaging in communication at the deepest level.

> We must build a new world, a far better world—one in which the eternal dignity of man is respected.
>
> —HARRY S. TRUMAN

Dialogue is a highly specialized form of discussion that imposes a rigorous discipline on participants. When dialogue is done skillfully, the results are extraordinary: stereotypes dissolve, mistrust is overcome, mutual understanding is achieved, a common ground for new insights is established, new perspectives are discovered, new levels of creativity are reached. Ultimately, the bonds of the community are strengthened.

DIALOGUE *Versus* DEBATE

Dialogue and debate are opposites. The purpose of debate is to win an argument, to vanquish an opponent. In dialogue, everyone wins. The worst possible way of gaining mutual understanding is to win debating points at the expense of others.

In a debate, we assume there are two opposing views; in dialogue, we assume that many people have pieces of the answer and together we can find a solution. In a debate, participants attempt to prove the other side wrong; in dialogue, participants work together toward common understanding. In a debate, people listen to find flaws and make counter-arguments; in a dialogue, they listen to understand. In a debate, we defend assumptions as truths; in a dialogue, we reveal assumptions for reevaluation. A debate is about winning; a dialogue is about exploring common ground.

> Short words **are best** and the old words when short are **best of all.**
>
> —WINSTON CHURCHILL

> When angry, count to ten before you speak; if very angry, one hundred.
>
> —THOMAS JEFFERSON

Strategies for Successful Dialogue

- Check for the presence of all three core requirements of dialogue: equality, empathic listening, identification of assumptions.
- Minimize the level of mistrust before pursuing practical objectives.

- Focus on common interests, not divisive ones.
- Use specific cases to raise general issues.
- Build trust before addressing issues.

Why use dialogue? Because it builds trust. Dialogue helps different groups to become more familiar and comfortable with each other. Cooperation develops naturally; people develop a sense of identity with those with whom they share community. Many of the strategies for successful dialogue may improve the quality of discussions and relationships between people in a variety of contexts where people come together to discuss issues of common interest.

There are numerous forums for conversation in the world today, including new ways of using computers to discuss and consult with others. At the same time, we are witnessing the revival of traditions such as the philosopher's café and the conversational salon. But first, let's look at that uniquely American form of discussion, the talk show:

"Here's Yetta—on the air at age 92" (*The Province*)
NEW YORK—It's 8:39 a.m. and the tape is rolling. The theme music fades. The host, in a bright-purple skirt and blouse . . . looks into the camera. She smiles.

"Good morning, everyone," she says. "This is Residents Update, and I'm your host, Yetta Bauer."

Talk-show fans would recognize the setup. It's the same one that Johnny uses. And David. And Arsenio. But the host is 92. And she broadcasts from a geriatric centre. . . . Yetta Bauer is the oldest talk-show host in the U.S. . . . Even as she waited to go on for the first time, she wondered why. "I was plenty nervous, so I hid a piece of paper on my lap with the questions. But it went fine."

Her first guest was a nurse's aide. Since then, she has interviewed an additional 34 employees and three residents. . . . Last July, a tabloid published her photo and a brief story calling her the world's oldest talk-show host. A couple of days later, David Letterman called. A week later, she was taken in a limo to his show, where she was introduced and received a wild ovation and a drum roll. . . . Letterman asked her how often she interviewed someone.

"When I feel like it," she said. Letterman cracked up. Bauer has a couple of rules. She never asks anyone's age—"it's no one's business"—and doesn't let guests criticize the nursing home. . . .

"The amazing thing," says Bauer "is not that I never knew I had this talent, if it is a talent. The amazing thing is it didn't show until I was so old. That's what I want other people to think about."

THE PHILOSOPHER'S CAFÉ

The world is witnessing the rebirth of a tradition of dialogue that dates back to the Greeks. Dr. Yosef Wosk of Simon Fraser University has just received the Order of British Columbia for his work in reviving the philosopher's café.

According to Dr. Wosk, "A philosopher's café provides an intellectual evening that involves high-level public conversations that break down barriers that have traditionally fenced off institutions of higher learning. Many of the participants are mature people at a stage of their life when they have time to explore philosophical issues and questions that they didn't have the luxury for earlier in their lives. They appreciate the challenge of deeper thinking and richer meaning and anything goes—religion, politics—you name it."

Today's movement caught fire in Paris in 1992 when the Café des Phares began holding *cafésphilo*. The sessions must have quenched a thirst for intellectual discourse, because they quickly spread throughout France. Philosopher's cafés are now popular across continental Europe, the United Kingdom, and North America. The rebirth of the café movement came about because of the aging population, the hunger for meaningful conversation, and the easy access to information and knowledge.

At a philosopher's café, a group of people come together in a public forum over food and drink to share their views. The café begins with an introduction to a topic—the person moderating the discussion may be a university or college instructor who finds it refreshing to leave the ivory tower behind and swap ideas with the general public. The moderator may play many roles, such as setting the topic and doing background research. The moderator should know the community, be sensitive to the venue and, above all, keep people on topic and prevent anyone from monopolizing the discussion.

> The heart of the fool is in his mouth, but the mouth of a wise man is in his heart.
>
> —BENJAMIN FRANKLIN

In the modern world, experience is mediated much of the time. Information is handed to us, and we are largely passive. The revival of the philosopher's café reflects our longing to create real discussion within an oasis of time. Similar in some ways to the concept of the Sabbath, it is time dedicated to talking together about things of meaning and value to us. With a lifetime of experience to share, people want to come together to use their minds and to speak out about things that really matter to them.

THE SALON

We've forgotten how to be together. Salons or salonlike gatherings are what humans have done since before recorded history. Our ancestors developed all kinds of rules and signals and etiquette that facilitated being together in groups. We've lost those social skills. We need to rediscover them, partly from other cultures and partly from our own fumbling, awkward experience.

—ERIC UTNE

Conversation is communion. It is basic to all endeavors and could possibly be the most important activity that human beings engage in. Through conversation we show respect, we communicate love, we inspire each other, we learn about others, we show our knowledge, we laugh, we cry, we live, we love, we learn— above all, we express ourselves.

The salon movement is currently experiencing a revival in communities across the Western world. This movement is more varied and generally less formal than the philosopher's café. It is reflected in the growing number of book clubs, professional work groups, and study circles springing up across North America during the past decade. As people turn off their television sets and their computers, get off their couches, and speak their minds, person-to-person, they are connecting with others in a truly human way.

> If you are way ahead with your head, you naturally are old-fashioned and regular in your daily life.
>
> —GERTRUDE STEIN, SALON HOST

History of the Salon

"To converse is human, to salon is divine."

—JAIDA N'HA SANDRA

The precursors of European salons were the symposia of Ancient Greece. Symposia, like salons, took place in private homes, in special rooms built for the purpose. During gatherings, six to eight guests ate, drank, and discussed everything from local gossip to politics and philosophy. Egalitarian in both subject and membership, the symposia brought together people from many occupations. This mix of people encouraged creative exchanges between members of different disciplines and kept the more powerful members of society in healthy contact with ordinary citizens. However, the symposia did not welcome women or foreigners.

The Ancient Romans imitated the symposia with their somewhat more decadent banquets. The Roman habit of welcoming artists and writers into their homes continued through the following centuries in Italy. French kings returned from wars in Italy, writers and scholars in tow, determined to set up their own literary circles. Wealthy wives of merchants and royal women residing away from court began to imitate this new fad. The result was the birth of the French salon. The seemingly innocuous nature of general conversation later helped salonists foment the French Revolution, because men were allowed to speak freely in conversational circles run by women.

Starting Your Own Salon

Anyone can organize a modern-day salon. If you would like to start one, extend an invitation to a dozen or so of your friends and friends' friends to attend a discussion group, and choose a topic for the evening. At the end of the first evening, spend time brainstorming a topic for the next session and then take a vote. Encourage people to invite friends and have fun speaking your mind.

If you decide to run the salon yourself, your personality and interests will determine the mood and goals of the salon. The number of people who attend will reflect how inspiring they find your vision. That is a lot of responsibility—and it means you determine the success—or failure—of the group.

> If everyone is thinking alike then somebody isn't thinking.
>
> —GEORGE S. PATTON

A better alternative is to extend an invitation to a variety of people to attend a discussion group concerning the development of a salon and to use the group assembled to develop the specific type of salon. The larger the group of people who are committed to the concept, the longer and more successful the salon will be. Here is the basic format:

- Hold a basic conversational salon, choosing one topic for each meeting.
- Choose one weekday evening per month and plan on meeting for two hours.
- Meet at the same person's home each time. Ideally, the home should be centrally located and offer a living room large enough to seat 12 people.
- Choose a topic for the first salon by brainstorming a list of subjects, then voting. Allow people to vote for as many topics as they like. When you've isolated one that everyone is interested in, you have found your topic.
- Choose someone to create a mailing or e-mail announcement to remind everyone of the place, time, and topic of the first salon meeting. This person can also act as facilitator for the initial

session. At the end of each meeting, ask for a volunteer to create the next announcement and facilitate the next salon.

- Collect a dollar per person, and give the proceeds to whomever is handling the mailing. Or use e-mail if everyone has an e-mail address.
- Bring potluck snacks and beverages, but don't plan any major meals.
- Encourage people to invite friends and add them to the mailing list.

SPEAKEASIES

During the Prohibition era (1920–1933), speakeasies sprang up everywhere. They were illegal bars, some of which were created for high society, but many were seedy joints. The old-time saloon had been almost exclusively male, but the new speakeasies welcomed women. Of social significance was the fact that men and women were drinking together. The homemade booze tasted so bad they mixed it with fruit juice to make the first "cocktail"—you guessed it—for women. Men had one foot on the old brass bar rail and now so did the women. The conversation must have shifted as significantly as the social structure. As for the term "speakeasy," it worked for the café society in the 1920s, and it's our message: speak easy! Here's our toast to you:

Remember that less is more.
Speak your mind.
May all your words be filled with courage.
Speak with kindness.
Listen with your heart.

𝔢 ASSIGNMENT

- What's on your mind?
- Where would you like to speak your mind?
- What would you like to say?
- Choose a forum, think about what you really want to say, and go for it.
- Why not start your own salon?
- At your next dinner party, put some topics in a hat and take turns drawing one. (Tell your guests you've just read a fabulous book where you got this idea.) Enjoy the discussions.

STEP

7

MENTALLY FIT
for LIFE

It is not enough to have a good mind.
The main thing is to use it well.

—RENÉ DESCARTES

B y now you may be wondering how you're going to put your creative juices to work. Maybe you've decided to pick up the flute, or you've signed up for a woodworking class. Some of you are learning French with CDs from the library, or starting a book club in your neighborhood. There are so many different ways to sharpen your brain.

Now is the time for you to create your own fitness program—one that you can develop as your mental fitness level rises and your interests change. We hope that, from now on, you will take any activity, any art, any skill, and go beyond where it has ever been before, to a new creative place. Push things to the edge. Then watch them become a reality that you live every day.

Having a mind that's fit doesn't mean that you learn algebra or physics easily, solve the world's political problems, or compose a rock symphony in an hour. It doesn't mean being the smartest in your group, always being right, never being in a bad mood. What it does mean is that you can control your thoughts, you can decide on the language you use, you can discard negative and disempowering beliefs, you

Just as your car runs more smoothly and requires less energy to go faster and farther when the wheels are in perfect alignment, you perform better when your thoughts, feelings, emotions, goals, and values are in balance.

—BRIAN TRACY

can make wise decisions. You can laugh more, and surround yourself with happy people. You can also choose to start a physical exercise program and stick to it. There are endless things we can do to become mentally fit.

In Step 7—a launching pad for your mental fitness program—we're going to give you strategies that you can pick and choose from. We'll give you dozens of suggestions to incorporate into a daily, weekly, monthly, or yearly plan for a healthy mind for the rest of your life.

The place to begin is to create your very own mental fitness program, one that stimulates and challenges and stretches you to new heights in everything you do. First, it is helpful to think about a mental fitness program in the way that you think about a physical fitness program. Here is how Dot Josey, a mental fitness program participant in her 80s, described it:

Physical Fitness	*Mental Fitness*
Shake . . .	the cobwebs from your brain and start the thinking process.
Walk . . .	hand in hand, communicating effectively, being understanding and nonjudgmental.
March . . .	to the beat of your own brainwaves.
Stretch . . .	your mind to expand creative thinking power.
Bend . . .	your ear, listen carefully, so your mind will absorb, clarify, then reflect.
Flex . . .	your mind to stimulate and learn new things.
Stand . . .	tall, enabling the mind to be alert and clear-thinking.

Raise . . .	your mind to be confident and assured.
Swing . . .	your mind to be able to approach problems from different angles.
Pull . . .	from your mind your experiences and imagination.
Push . . .	your mind to its capacity.
Breathe deeply . . .	and your mind relaxes, improving memory.
Rejuvenate . . .	your mind and you will solve difficult problems in a clear and concise manner.

Your monthly mental fitness program could look like this. Some activities, like crosswords, you might choose to do daily. Please note that this schedule does not include your physical fitness program. You can incorporate activities that you do by yourself, with your partner or a friend, in a group, at social events, and in community college or university classes. Pick and choose to create a personal mental exercise program.

Sunday	Monday	Tuesday	Wednesday	Thursday	Friday	Saturday
reflect	French tapes	crossword puzzle		art class		dinner party
read an inspiring book	French tapes		bridge club	art class	tour guide at the art gallery	try out a new recipe
visit a museum	French tapes	meditation class	write in your journal	art class		relax
take a long walk	French tapes	watch a documentary film	choir rehearsal	art class	tour guide at the art gallery	dinner party with your own salon

As Frederick Faust once said: "There is a giant asleep within every person. When the giant awakes, miracles happen." Do something different today—and begin to wake up that sleeping giant. When was the last time you memorized a poem? You can probably still recite some of the poems you memorized in school when you were a child. We don't *have* to memorize things any more, but now that you have the choice, it can be an extremely good exercise and very satisfying too.

Here are two stanzas (the first and last) from a famous poem by Robert Frost. Go to the library and do a little research about the poem and the author. Talk to your friends or colleagues about it instead of talking about the weather or the news. Learn a few lines and quote them. Then ask if they've ever heard of it. See what happens.

The Road Not Taken

Two roads diverged in a yellow wood,
And sorry I could not travel both
And be one traveler, long I stood
And looked down one as far as I could
To where it bent in the undergrowth; . . .

I shall be telling this with a sigh
Somewhere ages and ages hence:
Two roads diverged in a wood, and I—
I took the one less traveled by,
And that has made all the difference.

THE ROLE *of* HUMOR

Take time out for humor. As Gene Cohen says, "Humor is liberating. Use it liberally. It loosens the muscles and frees the mind to make new connections." Here's something to make you smile right now, a few notices written in English and posted in foreign countries:

Moscow hotel: *If this is your first visit to the USSR, you're welcome to it.*

Polish zoo: *Please do not feed the monkeys. If you have the right food, give it to the Zookeeper.*

Chinese hotel: *You are invited to take advantage of the maid.*

Practice telling jokes. Everyone loves a good joke. Most people say they heard a good joke the other day but can't remember the punch line. When you hear a good joke, make an effort to jot it down, learn it, and pass it on. Here's one from Ellen DeGeneres that's easy to learn:

You have to stay in shape. My grandmother, she started walking five miles a day when she was 60. She's 97 today and we don't know where the hell she is!

Look up the meaning of old sayings. Do you ever wonder where they originated? The cliché "Easier said than done" originated from something being more difficult to carry out than to contemplate. Sometimes it is "Sooner said than done," but now that wording appears more often in "No sooner said than done," which has quite a different meaning.

How about "easy as pie"? That's used to refer to a pleasantly uncomplicated task. It can't have to do with the making of pie, which is not easy; surely it derives from the eating of pie, much like the current "piece of cake." In 19th-century America, "pie" had the meaning of an easy match, a prize obtained without much effort, as in "Green dogs are pie for him [the raccoon]." This statement appeared in 1895 in the recreational magazine *Outing* and suggests the ancestry of the more recent "easy as pie."

Well, "for what it's worth," making sense of all that is good mental exercise, and it can be fun too. Did you ever "eat crow"? Have you ever had a "half-baked idea"? You might be thinking, "for crying out loud," this whole paragraph is "for the birds," or "for the life of me" I can't figure out what this is about! It's "not worth a hill of beans" anyway. I used to feel "footloose and fancy-free" until I started reading this page. Well, I think we've "come full circle." "A penny for your thoughts"? "Hats off" to James Rogers' *Dictionary of Clichés*.

If you can dream it, you can do it.

—WALT DISNEY

Read. Read. Read. Read out loud to your children, your partner, a friend, or just to yourself. Make a habit out of it. So says John Dryden, "We first make our habits, and then our habits make us." Start with 10 minutes a day. It's joyful.

Write. Write. Write. Write a book, write a love letter, write in your journal. Write a speech and then deliver it. Writing is one of the best mental activities for exploring your thoughts and improving memory. For many it is a lost art. Let's rekindle it. It's free and it's freeing.

Some like readin', some like writin', and some like 'rithmetic. Quizzes and puzzles come in a multitude of forms. We have introduced you to a variety of them. Pick the ones you are attracted to, which are quite likely the ones you do well on. What lies lurking in the others may, however, give your brain the best workout. Try them all—and don't give up too easily on the more difficult ones. Remember, you don't have to be an intellectual genius to have fun and get a good brain workout. The idea is not to test your intelligence; the idea is to give your brain a workout. Like physical fitness, if you start with a marathon, you're going to give up partway and never try again. The idea is to be challenged and have fun.

Some quizzes and puzzles are timed—some people like to run against the clock; some like to solve puzzles in a specified time. If you don't like that kind of pressure, don't do it. Some people like quizzes with lots of symbols, lots of numbers. Pick a variety of different types of quizzes, and don't shy away from the ones that seem too difficult. For "story puzzles," you need time to consider all the angles. Here's a sample story puzzle:

EXERCISE 1: **THE MAN IN THE ELEVATOR**

A man lives on the tenth floor of a building. Every day, he takes the elevator to the first floor to go to work or to go shopping. When he returns, he always takes the elevator to the seventh floor and then walks the remaining flights of stairs to his apartment on the tenth floor. Why does he do this? (See "Clues and Answers," page 245.)

A Note on the Puzzles

Try to solve them quickly. If you don't get the answer immediately, it does not reflect on your intelligence. You will find that the more puzzles you do, the easier they get or rather, the better you become at solving them.

In this book we avoid the word "test." For too many people it conjures up their school years and a grading system that wasn't always effective. But here's one exception: a little test for you—*our* kind of test.

> Accept the challenges so that you may feel the exhilaration of victory.
>
> —GEORGE S. PATTON

Life's a Test—You're Graded on a Curve

At age 4, success is . . . not peeing in your pants.

At age 12, success is . . . having friends.

At age 16, success is . . . having a driver's license.

At age 20, success is . . . having sex.

At age 35, success is . . . having money.

At age 50, success is . . . having money.

At age 60, success is . . . having sex.

At age 70, success is . . . having a driver's license.

At age 75, success is . . . having friends.

At age 80, success is . . . not peeing in your pants.

EXERCISE 2: THE MEN IN THE HOTEL

The **only** limits in one's life are **self-imposed.**

—DR. DENIS WAITLEY

Mr. Smith and Mr. Jones are two businessmen who book into the same hotel for the night. They are given adjacent rooms on the third floor. During the night, Mr. Smith sleeps soundly. However, despite being very tired Mr. Jones cannot fall asleep. He eventually phones Mr. Smith and falls asleep immediately after hanging up. Why should this be so? (See "Clues and Answers," page 246.)

Words have power. Increasing your vocabulary is a great mental activity, and so is building a stronger vocabulary—not just quantity, but quality. There are numerous books on the market that include words that build self-esteem, romantic words, words about feelings, about personalities, about character, about the roots of words—where they come from, where they're going. Try learning two new words a week and putting them into use—that's 104 new words a year. It makes you feel great. That's word power. Your mind will love you for it.

Speaking of roots: the word "trivia" comes from the Latin *tri-* and *via*, which mean "three streets." In ancient Roman times, at the intersection of three streets, city dwellers could peruse notices posted on a kiosk. They might be interested in the information, they might not; hence they were bits of "trivia."

And speaking of trivia: It's good for the brain too. Do you know what 111,111,111 X 111,111,111 equals?
It equals 12,345,678,987,654,321.
Go figure!

Do you know:

- The international telephone dialing code for Antarctica is 672.
- A full moon always rises at sunset.
- A penguin has sex only twice a year.
- A dragonfly has a lifespan of 24 hours.
- The female ferret is referred to as a jill.
- A group of kangaroos is called a mob.
- A group of owls is called a parliament.
- A group of unicorns is called a blessing.
- A group of ravens is called a murder.
- A group of officers is called a mess.

QUESTIONS *for* YOUR BRAIN

Gregory Stock has written what looks on the surface to be a simple little book titled *The Book of Questions*. Questions like "Would you eat a bowl of live cockroaches for a million dollars?" (Well, would you?) "Would you be willing to give up all television for the next five years if it would induce someone to provide for a thousand starving children in India?" "Given the choice of anyone in the world, whom would you want as your dinner guest? as your close friend? as your lover?"

This is not a book of trivia questions. As the author, Gregory Stock, points out, the questions are about you, about your values, beliefs, life, love, money, sex, integrity, generosity, pride, and death. The questions stimulate and challenge debate and discussion. You are encouraged to not simply answer yes or no, but to think about and explain your responses. Stock suggests using the questions as a point of departure, giving your imagination full rein as you play with the situation described. What a great way to spend an evening with friends. Getting to know them more deeply, having fun, and best of all, thinking about different things in different ways.

Self-talk   Interpret everything in a positive way. Look for good in every situation. Practice serendipity.

Positive visualization   See yourself as the person you want to be. Mentally rehearse the person you want to be.

Surround yourself with positive people   Being around critical, negative people is enough to sabotage all the good positive energy you are creating.

Learn every day   Feed your mind with books, magazines, tapes, and CDs loaded with positive messages. Just as you become what you read, you are what you think about.

Games shake up the brain   We know from Dr. Marian Diamond's research in the 1980s that playing bridge actually improves the immune system. Furthermore, there are dozens of excellent board games on the market. They are fun, social, stimulating, challenging, and good for your health.

Spend time in nature   "We need the tonic of wildness," said Thoreau, "to wade sometimes in marshes where the bittern and the meadow-hen lurk, and hear the booming of the snipe; to smell the whispering sedge where only some wilder and more solitary fowl builds her nest, and the mink crawls with its belly close to the ground." Rejuvenate your spirit by spending time in nature.

Watch out for stress   It can hamper your brain activity. Parts of the brain simply don't work as well under stress. It is very important to our mental abilities that we do whatever we can to reduce anxiety and stress in our lives. Stress is poison to the body and the brain. Take time out to relax and play. Yoga and meditation calm the mind. Make sure you get enough rest and sleep.

> What you think of yourself is much more important than what others think of you.
> —SENECA

A FUTURE FILLED *with* HOPE

If you've learned anything from this book, we hope it's the power you have within you to make positive decisions about becoming more mentally fit. We hope that your mind has been opened to its vast possibilities and you are going to get on the Mental Fitness Bandwagon from this day forward. We hope you will teach others what you have learned and thereby spread the good news that aging does not have to mean "losing it." We hope you will use this book as a guide to running your mind.

This is our personal challenge to you: tailor-make your mental fitness program daily, weekly, monthly, and yearly. Change it as you change yourself. But, above all, put it into practice. Make a commitment to yourself to become mentally fit for life, every day of your life. Make it fun and pass it on.

We're asking you to make a commitment, to embrace your age. To proudly welcome each new year as a milestone, savor the unique challenges that offer themselves, experience the richness, depth, and meaning in each phase and stage of your life with mental fitness running as a seamless thread through every moment, every hour, and every day.

> Make the most of yourself, for that is all there is of you.
>
> —RALPH WALDO EMERSON

To live each year, as Stephen Levine writes, "as if it were your last."

We ask you to bring a new sensitivity and awareness to the language you use, to sniff out any negative beliefs that hide behind the words. Change your words and beliefs to reflect hope and possibility, which will bring you closer to your dreams for the future. Develop your untapped well of creativity—to recognize that mature adulthood must be embraced for the opportunity it is to dip into the well of creativity. To make your life a true work of art. We challenge you to bring a positive mental attitude to everything you do and every relationship in your life; to find the opportunity and the joy that lurks behind every experience just waiting to be discovered.

We ask that you commit yourself to developing a memory that will astound your friends, that will capture the imagination of those who are important to you. We urge you to develop personal strategies for both learning and remembering the things that are important to you so that you never again need to fear memory loss. Sign up for a class, pursue something new, play a musical instrument, or take a language course. Choose your forum for speaking your mind. Join a university class, a book club, a philosopher's café, or a salon. If you can't locate one, start your own. Exercise mental, physical, emotional, and spiritual fitness every day of your life for the rest of your life, because *now* is the rest of your life.

We look forward to new research that validates what we believe about the possibilities for vital, healthy aging. We look forward to new research that validates the role of learning in healthy aging, that demonstrates what we can do, each one in his or her own unique way and style, to continue to develop our minds and our spirits well beyond what was achieved in the past. We look forward to the day when people of every age no longer marvel at the skills and talents and contributions of "older people," when there is no need for us to report that a woman in the U.K. has just received her degree at Cambridge at the age of 105, that a black man in the southern United States has learned to read at the age of 94, that a First Nations man in the Canadian Northwest Territories has just graduated from high school with his great-grandson.

We look forward to the day when we celebrate the accomplishments and successes of all people, no matter what their age, because we believe that anything is possible. Look over your shoulder—that day has just arrived.

🖉 HOW'S YOUR **MENTAL FITNESS NOW?**

Rate yourself on a scale of 1 to 10 (10 being the highest rating).

_____ 1. Confidence in your mental abilities
_____ 2. Setting and achieving goals
_____ 3. Willingness to take risks
_____ 4. Optimism
_____ 5. Creativity
_____ 6. Mental flexibility
_____ 7. Ability to learn new things
_____ 8. Memory
_____ 9. Ability to speak your mind clearly
_____ 10. Level of mental fitness

SELF-ASSESSMENT

Add up your score and rate yourself according to the following:

40–54   fair
55–69   good
70–84   very good
85–100 excellent

Go back to page 22 and compare your scores. As you continue to develop your mental fitness, we suggest that you retest yourself periodically. Keep shooting for 100!

AFTERWORD

Do not go gentle into that good night,
Old age should burn and rave at close of day;
Rage, rage against the dying of the light.

W hen Dylan Thomas wrote these lines in the mid-20th century, it was a call to arms for the aged, a romantic— almost quixotic—alarum to break the bonds of despair that the inevitable "close of day" held for us all. But all that he could offer was rage . . . heroic, desperate, but in the end futile rage. He was a creature of his time, and his plea, however inspiring, reflected the beliefs and wisdom of that time.

A half-century later, Sandra Cusack and Wendy Thompson have provided us with a document of liberation, a veritable Magna Carta for understanding and enjoying the second half of life. Their thinking represents a dramatic shift in the way we look at the process of maturation and aging. Based solidly in laboratory research, much of it from the Berkeley laboratory of Marian Diamond and her associates, *Mental Fitness for Life* introduces us to a fertile, dynamic period of life enriched by experience, yet also gifted by a plasticity—a potential for continual growth and enhancement of capacity—that could not even have been guessed at by the contemporary world of Dylan Thomas.

We are witnessing a powerful new way of thinking about the later years of life—at a time when life's envelope for most of us is expanding to and beyond the century mark. Suddenly, the years following retirement (a term increasingly archaic and inappropriate) have become decades, and these decades are now found to provide a rich soil appropriate for what can truly be considered a second lifetime.

The authors have provided us with a road map for exploring and realizing this newly minted epoch of our lifetime. This is an inspiring document, a "how to" book in the grand tradition, and one that can well serve us for the rest of our lives. The fact that we have the conscious ability to physically change our brains through the attitudes we adopt, the experiences we seek, and the skills we develop becomes the conceptual foundation for a new approach to life and a new zeitgeist. The authors have succeeded admirably in conveying the excitement of these new ideas—and solid, common-sense methods for the realization of their potential.

ARNOLD B. SCHEIBEL, M.D.
LOS ANGELES, CALIFORNIA

APPENDIX: CLUES and ANSWERS

INTRODUCTION

Answers to the Brain Teaser on page 36:
1. 116 years, from 1337 to 1453
2. Ecuador
3. From sheep and horses
4. November. The Russian calendar was 13 days behind ours.
5. Squirrel fur
6. The Latin name was Insularia Canaria—Island of the Dogs.
7. Albert. When he came to the throne in 1936, he respected the wish of his grandmother, Queen Victoria, that no future king should be called Albert.
8. Crimson
9. New Zealand
10. Duh!

STEP 1: GOAL SETTING

Mental Fitness Warm-Up
1. 1990 is one more than 1989
2. Yes

3. None—it was Noah.

4. Meat

5. Twelve

6. The operative word is "can," as in "tin can," and the solution is therefore self-evident.

7. The man was walking through a train tunnel and was almost at the end when he heard the whistle and spotted the train coming toward him. He therefore had to move forward, toward the train, so that he could jump clear safely.

8. A baseball player

STEP 2: **POWER THINKING**

Mental Fitness Warm-Up
Simply turn the block of stone over. So they did just that. And discovered that their grandparents had beaten them to it.

STEP 3: **CREATIVITY**

Warm-Up Exercises
EXERCISE 1: **The Mystery Paragraph**
There are no E's in the whole paragraph.

EXERCISE 2: **The River Problem**

Clue: The man uses a piece of rope. But how?

Answer: He stretches a long rope from point A to point B as shown in the diagram.

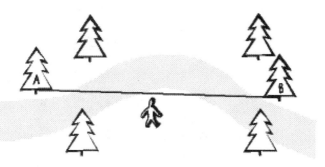

EXERCISE 3: **Blinded at Teatime**

Clues:

Q: Was there a flash of light or some other external occurrence?

A: No.

Q: Was the man physically normal?

A: Yes.

Q: Did something go into his eye because he was drinking the cup of tea?

A: Yes.

Answer: He had left his teaspoon in his cup of tea. When he raised the cup to drink, the teaspoon handle poked him in the eye, temporarily blinding him.

EXERCISE 4: **Connect the Dots**

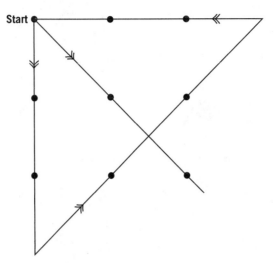

STEP 4: **POSITIVE MENTAL ATTITUDE**

EXERCISE 1: **Answers**

1. I'm overworked and underpaid
2. Circulating library
3. Don't overdo it
4. Gross injustice
5. Double pay
6. Man about town
7. Just in case
8. Forecast
9. Toronto
10. Getting it all together
11. Wedding ring
12. Backfire

EXERCISE 2: **The Miller's Daughter**

Clue: You have to think of a way whereby she could use the fact that she knows she will draw a black pebble to give a result that will indicate a white pebble. If that is too obscure, just remember that a double negative is a positive, and that should help.

Answers: Her best course of action is to take a stone from the bag and immediately drop it on the path. She can then say, "We can work out the color of the stone I selected by looking at the one that is left. If that is black, I must have selected the white stone."

Or she could say: "I feel so nervous . . . my hands are trembling too much for me to draw. Why don't you draw a stone, and the one that's left will be mine?" When he draws a black one, she can say, "The one that's left must be white."

STEP 5: **LEARNING AND MEMORY**

EXERCISE 1: **Answers**

1. Acorn	9. Idaho	17. Queen
2. Berlin	10. Jelly	18. Robin
3. Casablanca	11. Kew	19. Scouts
4. Delilah	12. Lama	20. Twister
5. Elk	13. Mars	21. Underwriter
6. Fats	14. Nelson	22. Ventriloquism
7. Goons	15. Ounce	23. Waterloo
8. Hogmanay	16. Pearl	24. Yachts

Rate your score:

10–12 fair   13–17 good   18–21 very good   22–24 excellent

EXERCISE 2: **The Lost Passenger**

Here are some clues:

Q: Did someone deliberately harm or abduct Billy?

A: No.

Q: Was his label removed in some way?

A: Yes.

Q: Was Billy a little boy?

A: No.

Q: Did Billy destroy the name tag?

A: Yes. (He ate it.)

Answer: Little Billy, as his name suggests, was a goat who unfortunately ate his label, so no one knew where he was supposed to go.

EXERCISE 3: **Weather Forecast**

Here are some clues:

Q: Was John some kind of weather expert?

A: No.

Q: Did he have some special knowledge or insight into the future?

A: No.

Q: Is this to do with timing?

A: Yes.

Answer: In 72 hours, it would be midnight again, so it could not be "bright and sunny."

STEP 6: **SPEAKING YOUR MIND**

EXERCISE: **The Man in the Painting**

Clue: This is a simple little riddle but it often causes consternation. If you get into a muddle with it then just divide the sentence into three parts:

- brothers and sisters have I none,
- but this man's father
- is my father's son

Now work backwards from the last statement.

Answer: It is the man's son in the painting. "My father's son" must be the man himself (since he had no brothers or sisters). Therefore, "this man's father is my father's son" becomes "this man's father is me." So the man in the picture is his son.

STEP 7: MENTALLY FIT FOR LIFE

EXERCISE 1: **The Man in the Elevator**

Here are some clues:

Q: Is there anything that he does between the seventh and tenth floors other than climb stairs?

A: No.

Q: If he had someone else with him, would they both get out at the seventh floor and walk up to the tenth floor?

A: No.

Q: If he lived on the sixth floor, would he go up to the sixth floor in the elevator?

A: Yes.

Q: If he lived in a different block of apartments in a different country but still on the tenth floor, would he still get out on the seventh floor when going up?

A: Most probably yes.

Answer: The man is a dwarf. He can reach the button in the elevator for the first floor, but he cannot reach the button for the tenth floor. The seventh floor button is the highest he can reach.

EXERCISE 2: **The Men in the Hotel**

Clues:

Q: Was there something happening in Mr. Smith's room that was preventing Mr. Jones from sleeping?

A: Yes.

Q: Was it a noise?

A: Yes.

Q: Did they speak for long on the phone?

A: No.

Answer: Mr. Jones could not sleep because Mr. Smith was snoring. His phone call awoke Mr. Smith and stopped him snoring long enough for Mr. Jones to get to sleep.

BIBLIOGRAPHY

INTRODUCTION *and* STEP 1: GOAL SETTING

Abrahams, J.P., W.J. Hoyer, M.F. Elias, and B. Bradigan. (1975). Gerontological research in psychology published in the *Journal of Gerontology* 1963–1974: Perspectives and progress. *Journal of Gerontology* 30(6): 668–73.

Brady, Michael E. (1984). Demographic and educational correlates of self-reported learning among older students. *Educational Gerontology* 10(1–2): 25–38.

Brain Boost. *Prevention,* August 1994: 28.

Bridges, W. (1991). *Managing Transitions: Making the Most of Change.* New York: Addison-Wesley.

Bromley, D.B. (1990). *Behavioural Gerontology: Central Issues in the Psychology of Ageing.* New York: John Wiley.

Burnham, P.W. (1994). *Life's Third Act: Taking Control of Your Mature Years.* New York: MasterMedia Ltd.

Burnside, I. (1993). Healthy older women—In spite of it all. *Journal of Women and Aging* 5(3–4): 9–24.

Chopra, D. (1990). *Quantum Healing.* New York: Bantam: 228, 229, 243.

———. (1991). *Creating Health: How to Wake up the Body's Intelligence.* Boston: Houghton-Mifflin: 95, 96.

———. (1991). *Unconditional Life: Discovering the Power to Fulfil Your Dreams.* New York: HarperCollins: 69, 70.

Clark, E., M.K. Gardner, and R.J. Howell. (1990). Changes in analogical reasoning in adulthood. *Experimental Aging Research* 16(2): 95–99.

Sister Constance. (1998). What does a 94-year-old have to look forward to: Only turning 95? Paper presented at the 27th Annual Scientific and Educational Meeting of the Canadian Association on Gerontology, Halifax, Nova Scotia, October 15–18.

Covey, Stephen R. (1994). "The Passion of Vision" in *First Things First*. New York: Simon & Schuster.

Cusack, S.A. (1995). Developing a lifelong learning program: Empowering seniors as leaders in lifelong learning. *Educational Gerontology* 21(4): 305–20.

Cusack, S.A., and W.J.A. Thompson. (1993). *Developing a Lifelong Learning Program for Seniors in New Westminster: A Unique Experience in Educational Leadership*. The Century House Association and Community Education, New Westminster School Board. Simon Fraser Union Board of Health, Ministry of Health, Province of British Columbia.

———. (1998). Mental fitness: Developing a vital aging society. *International Journal of Lifelong Education* 17(5): 307–17.

———. (1999). *Leadership for Older Adults: Aging with Purpose and Passion*. Philadelphia, Pa.: Brunner-Mazel.

Edwards, T. (ed.). (1961). *New Dictionary of Thoughts: A Cyclopedia of Quotations*. New York: Standard Book Company.

Featherman, D.L., J. Smith, and J.G. Peterson. (1990). Successful aging in a post-retired society. In P.B. Baltes and M.M. Baltes (eds.), *Successful Aging: Perspectives from the Behavioural Sciences*. New York: Cambridge University Press: 50–93.

Friedan, B. (1994). *The Fountain of Age*. New York: Simon & Schuster.

Goff, K. (1993). Creativity and life satisfaction of older adults. *Educational Gerontology* 19(3): 241–50.

Golden, D., and Alexander Golden. (1994). Building a better brain. *Life*, July: 63–72.

Goldman, R., R. Klatz, and L. Berger. (1999). *Brain Fitness: Anti-aging Strategies for Achieving Super Mind Power*. New York: Doubleday.

Hooker, K., and I.C. Siegler. (1993). Life goals, satisfaction, and self-rated health: Preliminary findings. *Experimental Aging Research* 19: 97–110.

Hoyer, W.L., C.L. Raskins, and J.P. Abrahams. (1984). Research practices in the psychology of aging: A survey of research published in the *Journal of Gerontology*, 1975–1982. *Journal of Gerontology* 39(1): 44–48.

Kaufman, S.R. (1993). Reflections on "The Ageless Self." *Generations* 7(2): 13–16.

Kerschener, H. (1994). The White House Conference on Aging Focus Group Project. *Gerontology News: Newsletter of the Gerontology Society of America*, December: 4.

Langer, E. (1993). *Mindfulness*. New York: Addison-Wesley.

———. (1997). *The Power of Mindful Learning*. New York: Addison-Wesley.

Lapierre, S., and L. Bouffard. (1992). Motivational goal objects in later life. *International Journal of Aging and Human Development* 36(4): 279–92.

Lapierre, S., L. Bouffard, and E. Bastin. (1997). Personal goals and subjective well-being in later life. *International Journal of Aging and Human Development* 45(4): 287–303.

Leirer, V.O., D.G. Morrow, J.I. Sheikh, and G.M. Pariante. (1990). Memory skills elders want to improve. *Experimental Aging Research* 16(3): 155–58.

Lewis, J. (1981). *Something Hidden: A Biography of Wilder Penfield.* Toronto: Doubleday.

Northrup, C. (1994). *Women's Bodies: Women's Wisdom.* New York: Bantam Books.

Okun, M.A., W.A. Stock, and R.E. Covey. (1983). Assessing the effects of older adult education on subjective well-being. *Educational Gerontology:* 523–26.

Rapkin, B.D., and K. Fischer. (1992). Framing the construct of life satisfaction in terms of older adults' personal goals. *Psychology and Aging* 7(1): 138–49.

Salthouse, T.A., S. Legg, R. Palmon, and D. Mitchell. (1990). Memory factors in age-related differences in simple reasoning. *Psychology and Aging* 5(1): 9–15.

Scheibel, A. (1995). Challenging the brain to stay in shape. *The Older Learner: Quarterly Newsletter of the Older Adult Education Network of the American Society on Aging* 3(1): 1, 8.

Seagull, S. (1995). Mind Your Mind: Workshops for Mental Fitness. *The Older Learner: Quarterly Newsletter of the Older Adult Education Network of the American Society on Aging* 3(1): 4.

Walsh, P.B. (1983). *Growing Through Time: An Introduction to Adult Development.* Monterey, Calif.: Brooks/Cole.

Wass, H., and H. Olenjik. (1983). An analysis and evaluation of research in cognition and learning among older adults. *Educational Gerontology* 9: 323–27.

STEP 2: POWER THINKING

Cusack, S.A., and W.J.A. Thompson. (1999). *Leadership for Older Adults: Aging with Purpose and Passion.* Philadelphia, Pa.: Brunner-Mazel.

Levy, B.R. (1999). The inner self of the Japanese elderly: A defense against negative stereotypes of aging. *International Journal of Aging and Human Development* 48(2): 131–44.

———. (2001). Eradication of ageism requires addressing the enemy within. *The Gerontologist* 41(5): 578–79.

McHugh, K.E. (2000). "Ageless self"? Emplacement of identities in Sun Belt retirement communities. *Journal of Aging Studies* 14(1): 103–15.

Minichiello, V., J. Browne, and H. Kendig. (2000). Perceptions and consequences of ageism: Views of older people. *Ageing and Society* 20(3): 253–78.

Palmore, E.P. (2001). The Ageism Survey: First findings. *The Gerontologist* 41(5): 572–75.

Robbins, A. (1992). *Awaken the Giant Within.* New York: Fireside.

Ulmer, M. (1999). A Modest Proposal for the Aged. *National Post,* July 5.

STEP 3: **CREATIVITY**

Brett, P. (1999). Creativity and healthy aging: Charting the directions for research. *The Older Learner* 7(3): 1, 6.

Buzan, T. (1994). *Buzan's Book of Genius*. New York: Random House.

Coghill, J. (1999). Elders and theatre arts: Finding meaning in the new millennium. *The Older Learner* 7(3): 4, 5.

Cohen, G.D. (2001). *The Creative Age: Awakening Human Potential in the Second Half of Life*. New York: Quill.

Cohen, G., and A. Terry. (2000). C=me2: The creativity equation that could change your life. *Modern Maturity* 43(2): 32–37.

Edel, L. (1985). Artist in old age. *Hastings Center Report* 15(2): 38–44.

Fisher, B.J., and D.K. Specht. (1999). Successful aging and creativity in later life. *Journal of Aging Studies* 13(4): 457–72.

Kastenbaum, R. (1991). Serious play and infinite limits. *Generations*, Spring: 6.

Ritchie, E. (1994). Who, me? Aging? *Ageing International* 2(4): 27–32.

Romaniuk, J.D., and M. Romaniuk. (1981). Creativity across the lifespan: A measurement perspective. *Human Development* 24(6): 366–81.

Sark. (1991). *A Creative Companion: How to Free Your Creative Spirit*. Berkeley, Calif.: Celestial Arts.

Spencer, M.J. (1996). *Life Arts Experiences: Their Impact on Health and Wellness*. A work in progress. Hospital Audiences, Inc.

Vance, M., and D. Deacon. (1995). *Think Out of the Box*. Franklin Lakes, N.J.: Career Press.

STEP 4: **POSITIVE MENTAL ATTITUDE**

Baltes, P. (2001). A lifespan view of development. Paper presented at a symposium, "Longevity and Healthy Aging." 17th Meeting of the International Association of Gerontology, Vancouver, Canada. July 1–6.

Buzan, T. (1994). *Buzan's Book of Genius*. New York: Random House.

Collins, C. (2001). The healthy brain: An interview with researcher and teacher, Marian Diamond. *The Older Learner* 9(3).

Cusack, S.A, W.J.A. Thompson, and M.E. Rogers. (2003). *Mental Fitness for Life: The Impact of an 8-week Mental Fitness Program on Mental Fitness, Self-Esteem, and Depression*. (submitted).

Glass, T.A., C.M. deLeon, R.A. Marottoli, and L.F. Berkman. (1999). Population based study of social and productive activities as predictors of survival among elderly Americans. *British Medical Journal* 319(7208): 478–83.

Lewinsohn, P.M., J.R. Seeley, R.E. Roberts, and N.B. Allen. (1997). Center for Epidemiologic Studies Depression Scale (CES-D) as a screening instrument for depression among community-residing older adults. *Psychology and Aging* 12(2): 277–87.

Northrup, C. (1994). *Women's Bodies: Women's Wisdom*. New York.: Bantam Books.

Nussbaum, P.D. (2001). Do brain studies point the way to a "learning vaccine"? *Aging Today* 11(6): 1.

Robins, R.W., H.M. Hendin, K.H. Trzesniewski. (2001). Measuring global self-esteem: Construct validation of a single-item measure and the Rosenberg Self-Esteem Scale. *Personality and Social Psychology Bulletin* 27(2): 151–61.

Schulz, R., J. Bookwala, J.E. Knapp, M. Scheier, and G.M. Williamson. (1996). Pessimism, age, and cancer mortality. *Psychology and Aging* 11(2): 304–309.

Segerstrom, S.C., S.E. Taylor, M.E. Kemeny, and J.K. Fahey. (1998). Optimism is associated with mood, coping, and immune change in response to stress. *Journal of Personality and Social Psychology* 6: 1646–55.

Seligman, M. (1998). *Learned Optimism*. New York: Simon & Schuster.

Snowdon, D. (2001). *Aging with Grace: What the Nun Study Teaches Us About How to Lead Longer, Healthier, and More Meaningful Lives*. New York: Bantam Books.

STEP 5: **MEMORY** *and* **LEARNING**

Abrahams, J.P., W.J. Hoyer, M.F. Elias, and B. Bradigan. (1975). Gerontological research in psychology published in the *Journal of Gerontology* 1963–1974: Perspectives and progress. *Journal of Gerontology* 30(6): 668–73.

Battersby, D. (1989). Ageing and lifelong learning in New Zealand. *Journal of Educational Gerontology* 4(1): 28–36.

Collins, C. (2001). The healthy brain: An interview with researcher and teacher, Marian Diamond. *The Older Learner* 9(3).

Cusack, S.A., and W.J.A. Thompson. (1999). *Leadership for Older Adults: Aging with Purpose and Passion*. Philadelphia, Pa.: Brunner-Mazel.

Glass, T.A., C.M. deLeon, R.A. Marottoli, and L.F. Berkman. (1999). Population based study of social and productive activities as predictors of survival among elderly Americans. *British Medical Journal* 319(7208): 478–83.

Highet, G. (1976). *The Immortal Profession*. New York: Weybright & Talley.

Hoyer, W.L., C.L. Raskins, and J.P. Abrahams. (1984). Research practices in the psychology of aging: A survey of research published in the *Journal of Gerontology*, 1975–1982. *Journal of Gerontology* 39(1): 44–48.

Leirer, V.O., D.G. Morrow, J.I. Sheikh, and G.M. Pariante. (1990). Memory skills elders want to improve. *Experimental Aging Research* 16(3): 155–58.

Nussbaum, P.D. (2001). Do brain studies point the way to a "learning vaccine"? *Aging Today* 11(6): 1.

Parrott, S. (2000). Long road to literacy: Texas man learned how to read at 98. *The Maui News*, February 9: C7.

Sloane, P., and D. MacHale (1994). *Great Lateral Thinking Puzzles*. New York: Sterling Publishing.

Snowdon, D. (2001). *Aging with Grace: What the Nun Study Teaches Us About How to Lead Longer, Healthier, and More Meaningful Lives*. New York: Bantam Books.

Thompson, W.J.A., and S.A. Cusack. (1991). *Flying High: A Guide to Shared Leadership in Retirement*. Vancouver, B.C.: Simon Fraser University.

STEP 6: SPEAKING *Your* MIND

Allen, F.L. (1931). *Only Yesterday: An Informal History of the 1920's*. New York: Harper & Row.

Battersby, D. (1987). From andragogy to gerogogy. *Journal of Educational Gerontology* 2(1): 4–10.

Behr, E. (1996). *Prohibition and the Thirteen Years That Changed America*. New York: Arcade Publishing.

Fishman, A. (2001). Generational targeted marketing. Paper presented at a symposium, "The Unretirement Trend and Lifelong Learning." First Joint Conference of the American Society on Aging and the National Council on the Aging, New Orleans, Louisiana, March 8–11.

Garr, A. (2001). When communication is an illusion. *Vancouver Sun*, May 19: E2.

Sandra, J.N., J. Spayde, and the editors of the *Utne Reader*. (2001). *Salons: The Joy of Conversation*. Gabriola, B.C.: New Society.

Yankelovich, D. (1999). *The Magic of Dialogue: Transforming Conflict into Cooperation*. New York: Simon & Schuster.

COPYRIGHT ACKNOWLEDGMENTS

INDEX